My Life As A Diet: Understanding and Healing for Never-ending Dieters!

By
Maurice Horwitz

With a Foreword
By
Stephanie H. Abrams, MD, MS
Chair of the Obesity Task Force
of the North American Society of Pediatric
Gastroenterology, Hepatology, and Nutrition

MY LIFE AS A DIET:
UNDERSTANDING AND HEALING FOR NEVER-ENDING DIETERS!

By

Maurice Horwitz

Book design by Maurice Horwitz

DISCLAIMER – This book is designed to provide information and motivation to our readers in their pursuit for good health. It is sold with the understanding that the author and publisher are not engaged to render any type of medical, psychological, or any other kind of professional advice, either directly or indirectly. This book is not intended as a substitute for medical advice of physicians or mental health professionals. The reader should consult a physician in matters relating to his/her health and particularly with respect to any symptoms that may require diagnosis or medical attention.

Horwitz Publishing LLC books are available through Ingram Press, and available for order through Ingram Press Catalogue

Visit my website at www.mylifeasadiet.com

Printed in the United States of America

First Printing: March 2014

Horwitz Publishing, LLC

ISBN 978-1-62747-029-2
EBook ISBN 978-1-62747-030-8
LCN

Dedication

This book is lovingly dedicated to all never-ending dieters. Your exceptional drive and strength to achieve your goals put you in an incomparable class of your own. This book is my gift to you, to let you know that you are not alone, that you have a friend who truly understands and cares, but more importantly, to inspire you to unlock and live all of your dreams and aspirations that you so deserve.

Acknowledgements

I acknowledge with love and gratitude:

The entire Horwitz "Dynasty"! To my wonderful, loving extended family, thank you all for your love and support during the good times and the difficult.

To all of my dear friends, thank you for being my life's cheerleaders, for being an incredible loving support system, and for loving me unconditionally no matter what size I am. I also give you special thanks for your patience, encouragement, and love during my process of writing this book.

I gratefully acknowledge Tom Bird and Ramajon Cogan, whose programs and guidance allowed me to write this book, helping me to make one of my life's missions a reality.

A special acknowledgement to the Reverend Joette Waters, whose guidance and support helped me to heal myself, and who enthusiastically assisted me in clarifying the affirmations that I use and present in this book.

I thank you all of your guidance, support, and love.

Contents

Foreword

It takes years to become an obesity specialist. After medical school and residency, I completed a three-year fellowship in Pediatric Gastroenterology, Hepatology, and Nutrition. I then spent 3 years getting a Masters of Science in Clinical Research, while seeing patients and running scientific research funded by the National Institutes of Health. My research has focused on childhood obesity and nonalcoholic fatty liver disease (NAFLD), the most common chronic liver disease in the world. A subtype of NAFLD is called nonalcoholic steatohepatitis (NASH), which can lead to cirrhosis, liver transplant, and death. Why is NAFLD the most common liver disease? The answer is most likely because of the obesity epidemic in our country.

Many people ask me why I decided to become an obesity specialist, especially my colleagues. I see the bias amongst many of my colleagues when it comes to caring for obese patients. The feeling is that there is so many diseases that people get where they had no control over getting the disease (maybe because it was genetically-determined). The feeling is that obesity is the patient's "fault." I was raised in a family that instilled a fierce sense of fairness and fighting for what's right. Society being biased against obese individuals for their disease without taking responsibility for society's role in developing this health epidemic is not fair. I am an obesity specialist because I feel obligated to fight for fairness and to fight for those children suffering with low-self esteem and depression related to their weight status.

I remember as a young child, my father and I went to the car dealership with my uncle. My uncle was the first morbidly obese individual that I ever knew. It was the 1970s, and he was severely, morbidly obese before people really were. I remember standing outside while my uncle got in and out of a Lincoln Continental. We were trying to decide if, with his size, the steering wheel was too close to his chest to make it safe. The discussion was about how this was the only car he could fit in. Back then, it was rare to see an individual weigh more than 300 pounds, but now it is rather commonplace.

Two-thirds of adults in the United States are overweight or obese. According to the Center for Disease Control (CDC), the majority of people living in our country weigh too much. And, "weighing too much" is linked to the three leading killers in our nation: heart disease, cancer, and stroke. The definitions of "overweight" or "obese" were not determined based on cosmetic criteria, but rather on disease criteria. Syndrome X or Metabolic Syndrome is the constellation of diseases that the overweight individual start developing: hypertension, diabetes, NAFLD, large waist size, and high cholesterol -- all related to the patient's weight status. So, if it's normal in our country to weigh too much, why is this disease associated with feelings of bias, belittling, blame, and isolation?

Obesity is the largest health epidemic in the world. Yet, social constructs have led to the isolation of those battling this disease, especially for those who have had a lifelong battle with obesity. Finally, here is a book that serves as a companion to the life-long dieter! As an obesity-specialist, I am thrilled to have this tool for my patients, a spiritual guide to overcoming unhealthy life-long dieting patterns. At last, the reader will discover a comrade who understands and comforts. This book guides and empowers life-long dieters to discover their strength, ability, and courage. It is time for life-long dieters to unite, and this book is the perfect platform. Congratulations on your journey, past and present. It has prepared you for your new beginning. Cheers to your future as a happy, healthy individual who has overcome deep adversity with grace and strength.

To my uncle in my story above, congratulations Uncle Moe! You have written more than just a book! This guide will serve as a platform to destroy the isolation that has surrounded lifelong dieters. You are truly an inspiration.

Stephanie H. Abrams, MD, MS
Chair of the Obesity Task Force of the North American Society of Pediatric Gastroenterology, Hepatology, and Nutrition

Introduction

Diet, after diet, after diet! Never-ending diets! If you have been on the diet roller coaster for any period of time, or for your entire life like myself, you understand how frustrating and tiring it becomes to continually try diet after diet, looking for that special weight loss magic. But somehow, our strength and beliefs keep us moving forward to the next diet in our continued hope to find the one magic formula that will, once and for all, take care of our weight problem. If this is you, welcome home!

Like many of you, I have lived my life this way and it is exhausting. So many years of being obese with all the dieting severely affected my self-esteem and the very spirit of my being. A few years ago, I had an epiphany about "my life as a diet," and it made me realize that of one of my missions during my lifetime would be to write a book for the masses of never-ending dieters who are like myself. Due to other pressing priorities, I needed to put writing this book on the back burner, knowing that it was something that I would eventually accomplish.

Recently, I had to deal with a number of serious, life-threatening health crises within a short span of time. During the course of these medical traumas, I gained back a significant amount of weight that I had just lost in the prior year. While recovering from the last of these crises, I soul searched and realized that somehow, someway, I had to stop my insane behavior of weight gain and come to terms with myself once and for all. My fat was the symptom, and "I" was the real problem! I realized that I needed to learn how to deal with "me"! This harsh reality that was now surfacing finally made me stop looking at the "fat" problem after all these years, and to begin really looking at the "me" problem. I knew that I had to have a "healing" if I was going to live, and most importantly, be happy with myself in my life. Thus, I developed a plan for healing myself. In doing so, I knew that the time was now to move forward with writing my book and to share this healing plan for all never-ending dieters who are like myself.

What I share with you in this book is my total honest, gut-wrenching truth. I know and understand how lonely and troubling being fat is, as well as all the monumental struggles that come with never-ending dieting. I wanted to bare it all for you and let you to know from my candid sharing that you are not alone, that there is someone out there who truly understands and cares, and that there is hope in the scary, lonely world of being fat and never-ending diets.

To my readers, let me suggest that you read through this book once. Then reread it and begin your healing journey at a point in the book that you determine is right for you.

I truly hope that I inspire you to have the courage and commitment to work with the healing plan that I present to you in this book. If you are steadfast in your personal commitment and conviction with this plan, it is my wish that you will experience a magnificent healing of your own, that you will be happy with the beautiful person that you are no matter what you weigh, and ultimately unlock and live all of your dreams and aspirations.

Maurice Horwitz

Part One

Understanding

Chapter One

Why this book?
Why this title?

Welcome! I am glad that you found my book and are joining me. You will soon discover that you are not alone.

Perhaps one of the worst feelings that a never-ending dieter experiences is a sense of isolation and loneliness in what seems to be an endless and unconquerable battle to lose weight. It would be wonderful if we all could have a friend by our side to aid us in sustaining our equilibrium and drive to achieve our goals during the diet process. A friend who understands our plight, assists us with our efforts, and helps to keep us on track, particularly during those times when we stumble and begin our "stinking thinking" that we are once again losing another battle in our raging war on weight.

The main purpose of this book is to give you a friend. Through printed words, I want to provide you with understanding, warmth, nurturance, hope, and positive strokes that only a true friend who understands can give you. We are going to help each other.

In addition, the second section of this book is about healing. It contains the healing of specific human qualities for the never-ending dieter that is restorative to our well-being, and for discovering, or rediscovering, our true magnificence and the realization of the amazing individuals that we truly are.

There are millions of overweight and obese people in the world, most in the United States. The latest statistics show that sixty-nine percent, or two-thirds of the adults in the United States are either overweight or obese. Childhood obesity has more than doubled since the 1970s. Over one hundred million people in the United States diet each year, typically making four or five diet attempts during the year period. The annual revenue of the U.S. weight loss market in 2010 was $60.9 billion, and the 2013 weight loss market revenues are estimated to reach nearly $67 billion! The numbers speak for themselves. We are definitely not alone, and there are a huge number of us never-ending dieters out there.

This book is not going to give you a new diet, or tell you what you should or should not eat. There are enough diet books on the market to last to infinity. It is a sharing of self-truths and knowledge from someone who truly cares, sincerely understands, and wants to help you, the never-ending dieters. We are way past due for being happy with ourselves no matter what we weigh, and living life to its fullest. The time is now!

WHY THIS TITLE?

Listening to a radio talk show as I was driving to work one morning, the host was discussing the degree of happiness and satisfaction that individuals experience in their lives. The host then asked, "If you could describe your life in five words or less, what would those words be? How do you feel about this phrase that describes your life?" In the blink of an eye, the breath left my body and I had to pull my car into a nearby parking lot. I sat there in a state of emotional collapse. The five words that I used to describe my life were, "My life as a diet!"

I was really in disbelief that I was actually describing my life as a diet. There were tears in my eyes and the reality of these words hit me hard. The truth hurts, and this was my absolute truth. I didn't want to accept it, but those were the words that came to me.

Since early childhood, I was always trying to conquer my being fat by endlessly searching for that miracle diet, that magic pill, the latest hot diet book, or the newest weight loss methods to lose weight. Fat was my enemy, and diets were my friends.

Yes, I had a career. Yes, I had a loving family. Yes, I had friends and a social life. I had my avocations that brought me great pleasure, and I did some traveling to see the world. But the bottom line for me is that my life had been lived as a diet and I needed to accept this truth.

Even today, as I write this book, I am still dieting to lose weight. The difference for me now is that with the acceptance of those five words describing my life came the certainty that I was not alone and that a community of people like myself existed, a community of like-minded, never-ending dieters who could join forces and help one another to achieve their goals, whatever those goals may be. Whether your brass ring is to lose five pounds, a hundred pounds, or to simply accept yourself to be healthy at a certain weight, united we stand. It is our birthright to be happy no matter what we weigh.

Throughout my life as a never-ending dieter, I have met and talked with hundreds of individuals who were dieting to lose weight. I discussed the problems and issues that they thought contributed to making them fat, and keeping them that way. Through my impromptu discussions about being overweight, I acquired a wealth of insights. Additionally, I had also achieved considerable personal growth through counseling. But nothing, absolutely nothing, speaks greater than walking the walk and talking the talk of a never-ending dieter. I know you agree that unless you have lived in our skin, the skin of a never-ending dieter, you will not understand us.

All of the above experiences melded together for me. I knew that I had to write a book to reach out to the multitudes of people like myself. This was my calling, my responsibility to proclaim, "Here I am! I am like you! You are not alone! Together, we can help each other! We are not alone!"

This book is meant to be your twenty-four-hour friend, and to be reread as often as needed. It is your companion to take with you wherever you go, and actively used during your good times, as well as the bad. Through the thought processes garnered from my experiences, knowledge, and insights, I hope that you will attain some of the understanding and healing that you desire to help you achieve your goals. Tools that are personal insights and knowledge that you already possess, but which may be in need of a little nudge to resurface for your continuous use.

Ultimately, I hope to aid each of you in reestablishing your self-worth, to deal openly with your inner conflicts and anxieties, and, most importantly, to help you achieve your goals, whatever they may be.

If this book helps even one person, I will consider it a success. I hope that person is YOU!

Chapter Two

Why Me?

*T*he one thing in my life that I know for sure is how to diet! In fact, I consider myself a diet expert, probably like most of you do as well. Looking for that magic diet to take me from fat to thin has always been my primary focus in life. It makes me sad to admit this, but it is true.

To demonstrate this great expertise that I declare to possess, here is but a sample of some of the many diets that I have attempted in my life, and why I understand never-ending dieters in their quest to lose weight. If you have been on any of these diets, medical interventions, or other weight loss methods at least once, if not numerous times like myself, we understand each other:

- Using the first commercial meal replacements marketed for weight loss, Metrecal and Sego, in the early 1960s
- Joining the TOPS® (Take Off Pounds Sensibly) organization for weight loss
- At age twelve, taken to a "weight loss specialist" and given injections of cow placenta

- Taking the diet pill tenuate dosepan prescribed by my primary care physician when I was a mere fourteen years of age
- Joining a gym specifically to lose weight with exercise
- Medically supervised starvation while in a hospital (at age seventeen, a medical research patient on obesity for three months)
- Grapefruit and egg diet
- Hypnosis (two times)
- Taking the drug preludin to lose weight
- Weight Watchers® (age twenty-three, the third time I joined, I lost 140 pounds in a year, but gained it all back and more – over the years I rejoined countless times. It's still a great program!)
- The Stillman Diet©
- The Scarsdale Diet©
- The Atkins Diet® (numerous times)
- Overeaters Anonymous® (in and out of meetings over the years)
- Rice Diet Program
  Durham, North Carolina
- Structure House Program
  Durham, North Carolina (Great program!)
- The National Institute of Fitness,
  St. George, Utah
- The Beverly Hills Diet©
- Pineapple enzymes
- Optifast® (three different times)

- Going to a treatment center for compulsive overeating
- Phen–fen (lost 140 pounds in six months — you know what happened after that!)
- Individual nutritional counseling with a dietician
- Optimum Health Institute® (OHI), Austin, Texas
- Cabbage soup diet
- Sugar Busters® diet
- Calorie counting (many times)
- Carb counting
- Fat gram counting
- Slim-Fast®
- Dr. Sears Zone Diet®
- The South Beach Diet®
- Medifast®
- Televised infomercial diet program
- Yet another medically supervised liquid protein diet at a local hospital in Houston, Texas (two times)
- Nutrisystem®
- Lap band surgery
- Quick Weight Loss Center® diet
- Using diuretics and/or laxatives
- Raspberry ketones
- Saffron extract for appetite suppression
- Freshly prepared calorie-restricted meals delivered to my home biweekly
- The perfectionism of dieting...I know the exasperating feeling of being on a diet, and then after two successful meals, or a

few successful days or weeks on the diet,
eating something off the plan and letting
this one instance revert me into my old
eating patterns.
- AD INFINITUM...

The list could go on, but you can see, feel, and
understand my diet history. It is overwhelming! I am
sure there are other diets not mentioned above that
you have tried, and it would be a safe bet for me that I
have tried that diet too.

In addition to my understanding never-ending
dieting, and perhaps more important to this
discussion, is my deep, empathetic comprehension of
what it means to be and live fat. As a child, I was fat.
Through puberty, I was fat. As an adult, I was fat. I
have lived and breathed fat. I have laughed and cried
(a lot) fat. I have been down every path in life fat, and
I sincerely understand the unique mechanics behind
the fat mind and body. I have experienced the miseries
and the horror of the continual battle, the endless
dieting that exhaust the very soul of my being. It has,
and continues to be, a very difficult struggle, creating
great wounds that hurt, really hurt. So as I shared my
diet history with you, I now reveal to you my
understanding of living fat:

- I have lost and gained hundreds upon
hundreds of the same pounds in my
lifetime.
- I have spent tens of thousands of dollars
in my pursuit of permanent weight loss.

- By age nineteen, I weighed over three hundred.
- At age forty-five, I weighed five hundred and five pounds.
- I know how it feels to lose twenty pounds in three weeks, then regain thirty pounds in the following four weeks.
- In my childhood, I remember the horrid, shameful feeling that I experienced when my classmates or other children I came in contact with exclaimed, "Look at fatso," or chanted, "Fatty, fatty two by four, can't get through the bathroom door!"
- In my teens, I remember how it felt to hide in my bedroom and devour bags of candy and/or packages of cookies that I had carefully hidden in my chest-of-drawers earlier in the day.
- I understand the heartbreak of not being invited to dances or other social outings when all of my peers were.
- I know the desperate action of retrieving packaged food from the trash that I had thrown away so I could finish eating it.
- I know the feeling of not being able to tie my shoes without a cardiac struggle.
- I know the feeling of a flushed face and pounding heart from climbing a single flight of stairs.
- I understand what it means to act ill, or make up another excuse to decline social

engagements since I did not want people to see me because of my weight.

- I know the degrading experience of having to shop in the specialty fat clothing stores, or buy through clothing catalogs so I do not have to deal with it in person.
- I understand the total embarrassment of ripping clothes due to the excess strain on the seams.
- I understand the devastating thought process of believing myself to be sexually inadequate because of my fat.
- In my teens and early adulthood, I knew what it meant to wake up at three in the morning and attack the contents in the refrigerator, or get dressed and go out in the dead of night to buy food to binge on.
- I understand the frustration and personal embarrassment of preparing to entertain friends and having to make a return trip to the grocery store a few hours before their arrival to buy more food and/or another dessert because I had eaten it.
- I know that commitment syndrome of starting that new diet tomorrow, but tomorrow never comes.
- I understand how It feels to have very loving but overly concerned family members who gave me pitying looks and constantly asked, "How's your weight?"

- I have experienced the embarrassment of getting stuck in a theater seat, or breaking lawn furniture.
- I understand the sheer horror of getting on an airplane and praying that there would be an open seat next to my assigned seat.
- I also understand coming to terms with the necessity of buying two seats on an airplane so I did not have to deal with the embarrassment of being asked to get off the plane, or told that I needed to buy a second seat for myself at that time.
- When traveling alone, I know the drill of ordering enough food for two people through a hotel's room service.
- I remember the sad feeling that I experienced while watching people active in sports wanting desperately to be a part of the activities.
- I know how it feels to be turned down for a job because I was fat.
- I know the fear of heart attack or stroke.
- I know the harsh reality that obesity is a major risk factor for cancer.
- I know the constant distress from knee pain and the effects that osteoarthritis have on my mobility and daily living.
- I understand the frustration and distress that my being fat created for my dear friends.

- I understand the terribly sad, disappointing feelings that I experienced when I was invited by friends to travel with them but had to say no because of my fat-related issues like my impaired mobility.
- I know the scary feeling of having a life expectancy much less than a man of a normal size.
- I understand how it feels to live vicariously through other people.
- I have lived the heartbreak of feeling unloved because I was fat.
- I understand defining myself by the number on the bathroom scale and how it influenced my daily living.
- I understand that self-loathing feeling upon seeing my reflection in a mirror.
- I understand the mental whippings of that critical voice that judges me so harshly because I am fat.
- I understand what it means to be ostracized, criticized, immobilized, compromised, and shamed for being fat.
- I totally understand the feeling of wanting to give up everything to wake up thin, with my compulsion to overeat gone from my life.
- I UNDERSTAND WHAT IT MEANS TO BE FAT!

So my life has been an epic story of dieting, with all the traumas and dramas that accompany this struggle.

I have lived with a "fat" mind with a total diet mentality. I know all of the frustrations, despair, guilt, fears, anger, anxiety, depression, insecurities, and craziness that being a never-ending dieter invites. I understand to the very core of my being that desperate, nonstop frantic feeling of wanting to give up everything, yes everything if only I could lose weight and keep it off.

Why have I written this book? I UNDERSTAND! I am not alone. You are not alone. We are not alone!

Chapter Three

Me, the Big C, a New Knee, and Cookies!

*I*n the prior chapter, I provided you with my "credentials of understanding" for never-ending dieters. Now I will go into more depth by sharing some very personal recent history with you that exhibits even more of my grasp on the human condition of being fat, using food as an escape mechanism, and never-ending dieting. Though difficult for me to share this, I believe that this story will strike a nerve with countless numbers of you.

I worked as an accountant with the United States Government for twenty-six years, and I was in major job burn-out mode during the final two years of my career. In addition, my physical and emotional health was failing during this period.

I suffered from severe osteoarthritis in both knees, caused by years of abuse from being obese. I had wanted to get my knees replaced, but the orthopedist said that I really needed to get below the three hundred pound mark to accommodate the hardware that was used for the knee replacement. Though attempt after attempt was made, I was never able to get to that weight threshold to have the replacements. I lived with constant knee pain. I had to use a cane, and at times when the pain was really bad I used a walker. I was feeling very old before my time. In addition, I had high blood pressure that remained at elevated levels even with medication therapy. I was a physical, emotional, and mental wreck of a man.

At this point in time my latest diet attempt was being on a liquid protein diet (yet once again) and it was short lived. My weight already in the high three hundreds was increasing with the nonstop binging that followed this latest diet effort. I didn't know where to turn, or what to do with myself. Had I been in the position before? Of course! But this time it was different. I knew that I must take radical actions to save my life once and for all, and get my mobility back with new knees.

In using the word "radical" (I admit that the following is very painful for me to share), I had lap band surgery three years earlier. I lost a mere thirty-five pounds by quickly learning how to eat around the inflated band. I returned to the surgeon to see if I could get a revision from the band to the gastric bypass. Due to a pulmonary embolus that I had a few months after my lap band surgery, the surgeon told me that I was no longer a candidate for another abdominal surgery like the bypass or the "new" gastric sleeve procedure. The door had been shut for me on this radical weight loss path.

There have been many times in my life when I have made crazy decisions based upon my need to lose weight. But this time was different. After many sleepless nights I knew what I had to do for myself. The decision was made. I was going to retire early from my job and make an extreme move to deal with my weight. I met with my brother and sister and told them my plan, that being, I was taking early retirement from my job and I was going to Durham, North Carolina, to participate in the Rice Diet Program. They were thrilled to hear my decision as they instinctively knew that if I did not do something extreme, I might not be around much longer.

The Rice Diet is a residential program that was based in Durham. Unfortunately, this program ceased its operations recently. Dr. Walter Kempner developed this diet in 1939 at the Duke University Medical Center for patients with high blood pressure and renal diseases. The outcomes for the patients following this diet were overwhelming, not only with lowering blood pressure and the reversal of kidney disease, but also the reversal of certain heart disease issues and diabetes. A surprising side effect from the diet was a very fast, significant weight loss. Word got out about the dramatic weight loss and the positive health effects from this diet. The Rice Diet Program became very popular and over the years helped thousands of patients to lose weight and to thrive with significantly better health. I happen to find out about this diet in 1980 from a close friend and knew instantly that I had to do this program. In 1981, I moved to Durham to be a participant on the Rice Diet, losing two hundred pounds in a year and going below the two-hundred pound weight mark for the second time in my adulthood. This was monumental and only one of the two occasions when I would go below the two-hundred-pound mark in my life, to date! Like many of us do after a large weight loss, I gained it all back, and more, within three years. The shame quotient that I lived with was mind-boggling.

But I knew in my heart that this time the Rice Diet would be my magic, or so I had convinced myself. I was much older, my life was at a different juncture than it was back in the 1980s, and in my heart I knew that it would be different for me this time. Just three months after making my decision, I took early retirement. Ten days later I was driving to Durham to begin my latest life transformation on the Rice Diet Program. Based on my maturity, necessity, and passionate commitment, this time would be my final transformation.

I began the Rice Diet Program weighing four hundred and twenty pounds. Thirteen months later, in the month of November, when I departed Durham for my hometown of Houston, Texas, I weighed two hundred eighty-two. I had lost one hundred and thirty-eight pounds in thirteen months that included an almost two-month weight plateau. I went from wearing a 5XL shirt to XL, and a size sixty-eight pants to a forty-eight. But the main triumph from my hard work, I was finally below the three-hundred-pound threshold. It was time to begin the knee replacement process.

The week after I arrived in Houston, I went to my orthopedist to discuss my first knee replacement and set a date for the surgery. During my appointment, I mentioned to the doctor that I had been experiencing some numbness in my left foot. Before moving forward with my right knee replacement the doctor wanted me to have an MRI of my lumbar spine just to make sure that there were no issues present that were causing this numbness and that could potentially have an effect on my knee replacement recovery process.

Two days later, I had an MRI of my lumbar spine. The radiologist, who happened to be my nephew, called me in to go over the test results. We sat down to look at the MRI and what followed would change my life, and my weight! Not only did I have stenosis of my lumbar spine (a narrowing that constricted the spinal column) that was causing my foot numbness, but during the MRI, the technician noticed a golf ball size shadow on my right kidney. My nephew showed me the MRI results on a computer screen and told me that I needed to look into this shadow on my kidney immediately. NOW!

To make a long story brief, I had additional tests, saw two oncologists, and both determined that I had cancerous tumor in my right kidney until proven otherwise. The bottom line: the tumor needed to come out. I had not exhibited any symptoms whatsoever, and by accident during this MRI, the cancer was discovered. It was at this time when I learned from the doctors the eye-opening fact that obesity is a major risk factor in developing cancer. It quickly became painfully obvious to me that my being fat was the main contributing risk factor of my developing this cancer.

The Big C! Cancer! Me? No, this couldn't be. This couldn't happen to me. This only happened to other people, not me! I was going to have a knee replacement, and now I was diagnosed with kidney cancer. Needless to say, I was devastated and completely overwhelmed. My family and friends kept telling me how lucky I was that it was discovered now and not a few months or years later when it might be too late to treat it.

But how would I endure this? I had lost my oldest sister Ruth, a magnificent lady who was the matriarch of our family, to a rare form of cancer just three years earlier. This wasn't happening to me. Our family had endured enough pain from my sister's cancer battle. Remembering the agony that my departed sister's children, grandchildren, and husband went through, as well as myself, my other sister, and my brothers haunted me to this day. Then two years after her death my oldest brother's wife was diagnosed with uterine cancer. Fortunately, it was caught in the early stages, she had successful surgery, and completed both chemotherapy and radiation treatments to prevent any further health problems or recurrences.

No more cancer would or could invade our family. Yet, now me! My brain would not stop its catastrophic thoughts. What if this happened? What if that occurred? What if...if...if? The tears began, until...

How did I handle this news, the tears? What any self-critical, very scared, never-ending dieter would do, I returned to food. All the hard work that I had done in Durham on the Rice Diet Program during the past year did not matter. All the wonderful changes to my body and overall health did not matter. All of the money that I had spent to get where I was now physically did not matter. Everything I had given up to lose weight and change my life to enable me to get back my mobility did not matter! I began eating to stop the tears and deal with the pain of the reality of my Big C. My medication, my drug of choice as they say, was food, and once again it became my best friend in the blink of an eye.

I clearly remember driving home after my appointment with the kidney surgeon having set the date for the surgery to remove the tumor, and if necessary remove my entire right kidney. Then magically, my "Mr. Hyde," who will be introduced to you in the next chapter, took the wheel and turned my car into a grocery store parking lot. Mr. Hyde parked the car and would soon begin food shopping for my cancer apocalypse. First stop, the cookie aisle.

Within the eight weeks from the discovery of the tumor to my surgery date, I gained forty pounds. A heavy sigh comes forth from me!

The surgery was a total success with only twenty percent of my right kidney needing to be removed with the cancerous tumor being totally encapsulated and contained. I was going to be okay and fortunately I did not need either chemotherapy or radiation. I was going to live! My prayers had been answered. I was one very lucky man.

But unfortunately, the eating did not stop. The habitual momentum was back in full force. During the recovery process I gained another ten pounds.

Move forward four short months, even with the recent weight gain of fifty pounds that took me over the three-hundred-pound surgical target level, I proceeded with my first knee replacement due to the extreme pain that I was continually experiencing from my right knee. Two surgeries within four months of each other! My successful knee replacement was followed with a month stay in a rehabilitation center. Somehow another twenty pounds appeared on my body during that summer, aided by the month of institutional food at the rehab facility. I was now up seventy plus pounds in eight months. Even with the great progress that I was experiencing with my knee replacement, the eating continued. I was out of control again. Of course the out-of-control eating was coupled with, you guessed it, intermittent diet attempts. Knowing that I was not supposed to gain weight with a knee replacement did not matter. I continued my crazy behavior and continued to eat.

In an effort to stop this insane behavior, I knew that I needed to get help. With rumors that the Rice Diet Program was closing in a few months, I returned to Durham in hopes to get myself back in control.

I participated on the Rice Diet for six weeks and due to the pending closure of the program moved to Structure House, another excellent residential diet program in Durham. The Wellspring at Structure House program offers a more realistic, all-encompassing approach to long-term weight control, albeit with a slower weight loss. I knew that this program would be a great bridge for my return home and would keep me centered and on the right track.

In my ten-week return stay to Durham, I lost thirty pounds between the two programs. Unfortunately, I was on the threshold of yet another health crisis that was rearing its ugly head. Upon standing or walking for more than a minute, numbness would start moving down from my waist level down into my lower extremities. I knew from the continued episodes of this new symptom that my lumbar spine stenosis, which had been diagnosed a year earlier with the MRI when my cancer had also been discovered, was once again acting up.

What followed? Another MRI. Then one month later I had laminectomy surgery on my lumbar spine. Five days after this surgery I began running a high fever that eventually led to the discovery of two dangerous, hospital-acquired infections that were present in my surgical incision. Even with heavy doses of extremely strong antibiotics that I began receiving, the infections were not getting any better. Just twelve days after the first surgery it was necessary for me to have yet another surgery to allow the surgeon to clean out my incision to accelerate the healing from these infections. I ended up being in the hospital for a month. This was followed by another month at home that included home nursing care visits and antibiotic IV infusions that I personally gave myself twice daily. I was in the midst of a medical nightmare. My message to you here: unless absolutely necessary, stay as far away from hospitals as humanly possible!

Within a twelve-month time frame I endured four major surgeries including a life-threatening infection. Enough was enough! I needed to heal, not only physically but also from the emotional stress that goes along with such health crises, or perhaps I should use the term health "opportunities" as a dear friend of mine refers.

While at home recovery from the infection I knew that I had to stop this insanity with food. I had to deal with this issue sanely, intelligently, and lovingly once and for all, whatever this would end up meaning for me. I was tired of feeling defeated. I was tired of the low self-esteem, the diets, and waiting for that magic number to appear on the bathroom scale before I could really be happy and live. Enough was enough!

So during this time I reflected upon all that I had been through in my life of dieting and dealing with being fat. I reflected on the good times and bad. I reviewed the diet programs that I had participated in and what I had learned. I reviewed my times in therapy over the years and the life events that had moved my soul to its core. I needed to face myself head on, with brutal honesty, to enable me to reach a pinnacle of forgiveness, self-acceptance, and true self-love once and for all. My focus was going to be on ME, not the fat!

My soul searching led me to some basics that I knew would work for me. In addition, I spoke with my spiritual mentor, a Science of the Mind practitioner who helped me on a path to further develop a method of healing that I used to start my climb to this new pinnacle of self-awareness and love. Instantly, it began to work, and continues to do so. This is a path of hope and healing that I will be sharing with you in the second part of this book.

But first, let me introduce you to my "Mr. Hyde"!

Chapter Four

Maurice and his Mr. Hyde

"It was on the moral side, and in my own person, that I learned to recognize the thorough and primitive duality of man; I saw that, of the two natures that contended in the field of my consciousness, even if I could rightly be said to be either, it was only because I was radically both..." Quote from, *The Strange Case of Dr. Jekyll and Mr. Hyde* by Robert Louis Stevenson

I once had a private discussion with one of my brothers about my eating habits and being overweight. My brother, who is five feet six, weighs one hundred thirty-five pounds, and who has no concept of what being fat or a never-ending dieter means, asked me point blank, "What happens to you that sets you off on a binge?" Without hesitation, I replied, "Something strange happens. Whether it is a problem or a situation that I am dealing with or that is plaguing my mind, a negative emotion that is harassing me, or during a period of boredom or loneliness, whatever it is, in the blink of an eye, my 'Mr. Hyde' emerges and my consciousness is now his."

So begins, "The Strange Case of Maurice and his Mr. Hyde!" So begins my binge process!

I went on to express to my brother that once Mr. Hyde is there, his momentum in securing food to eat is incredibly fast. Even if the choice of food that my Mr. Hyde prefers to eat at that particular moment is not available, he will find a way to make do with what is on hand. So a binge may be made of cookies and ice cream that Mr. Hyde purposefully seeks out, or the binge could also be made up of a chicken breast and salad that is readily accessible and on hand. But as it is poetically said of a rose, a binge, is a binge, is a binge! It does not matter what the type of food is eaten. Nor does the amount of food really matter. If the resulting behavior is uncontrolled, nonstop eating, it is a binge.

We all have our "demons," our own "Mr. Hyde," and they occur in each of us in different forms. No matter what metaphor we choose to call our demons, they are there in all of us. They are part of our being, of our consciousness. The crazy thing about this part of our inner self is that in actuality, it is the sum of our personal fears, anxieties, doubts, unhappiness, and the other undesirable forces in our psyche. These demons are the result of years of constant negative thinking, poor choices that we made, the bad habits we developed, and the resulting crazy behaviors that we continually practiced. Just like positive choices and behaviors that quickly become second nature to us, these negative choices and behaviors get stronger every time they are accessed and utilized for what we think is for our well-being. At least this is what our

Mr. Hyde wants us to believe. The more we use the "demons," the more we allow our fears to control us, and the quicker and easier they become to access. Our "demon" is definitely our coping mechanism for the negatives in life, and sometimes for celebratory positive events as well.

Notice that I used the term "choices" above. It is true that every second of every day we are making choices. No matter how small the choice is from choosing the clothes we will wear today to the major decisions like the purchase of a house, we are making choices constantly, both consciously and subconsciously. From my experience, the negative choices become much stronger as we continue to select them, and at the same time, these negative alternatives will become even harder to reverse.

The negative choices that might have taken longer to access years ago are now being accessed in that "blink of an eye," as I expressed to my brother. This "blink of an eye" access is due to the historical choices and practices that I constantly made when it came to handling my emotions and the uncomfortable situations in my life. When any of these issues surfaced, my Mr. Hyde would also surface and I would practice the irrational eating behaviors while being in this state of mind. Mr. Hyde's access eventually became instantaneous.

Our brain is an amazing organ with incredible power. Every emotion we have, every impulse or feeling, begins through the thoughts in our brain. When we make a choice or take action on a particular emotion, impulse, or feeling, we begin the creation of impressions in our brain that over time become the repeated habit of how we will respond to or deal with the same situations, emotions, or feelings when they return.

The same process also works through our thoughts regarding ourselves as being fat with our diet histories. The self-esteem issues, the hurts we have endured, and the diet "failures" that we believe we have experienced also become imprinted in our brains and feed our demons, that destructive part of our consciousness that lies within us. These destructive negatives are incredibly persuasive as we have all experienced. The good news is that they are reversible!

There is a saying by Albert Einstein that is frequently quoted in twelve-step recovery programs: "Insanity: doing the same thing over and over again and expecting different results." This is how I have operated throughout my life when it came to being fat and dieting. Like you, I have had successes, but I never fully allowed these successes and positive behaviors to leave their permanent impressions into my mind and create the incredible brainpower that results from these new imprints.

This is what the healing in this book is about. The healing is a practice of changing our thought patterns and attitudes. These changes in thoughts and attitude will materialize with devoted practice. Maybe, just maybe, this time we can triumph together by making peace with our demons by allowing them to coexist in harmony with our positive thoughts, harmony within our conscious and subconscious, thus resulting in a healthy state of mind that will lead us to great physical accomplishments. With the right focus, consistent work, and most importantly the desire to make the change we need to make within our minds thought processes, success and happiness will be at our fingertips. Let this exciting, life-changing journey begin!

Photo Gallery

The following are a series of photos of myself in
"My Life As A Diet" journey...

These photos show me from
one year of age in 1950,
through 2011, and the various
ups and downs with my
never-ending diets.

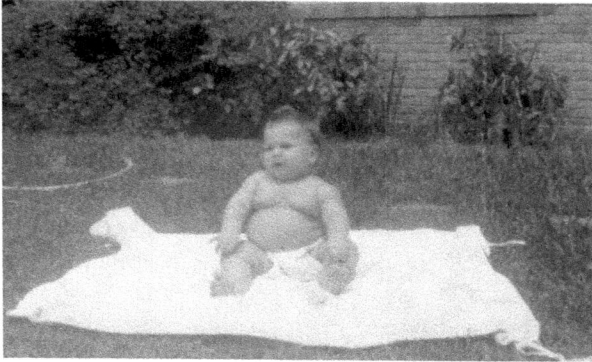

Year 1950, one year old (A big baby! – 42 pounds)

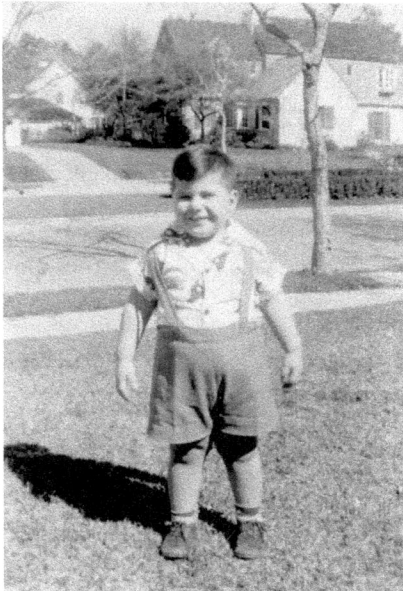

Year 1953, four years old

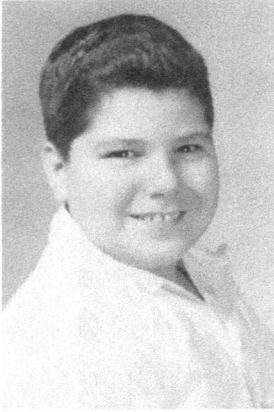

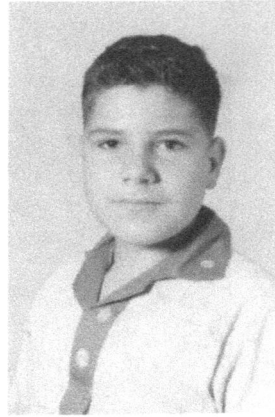

Year 1959, ten years old   Year 1960, eleven years old

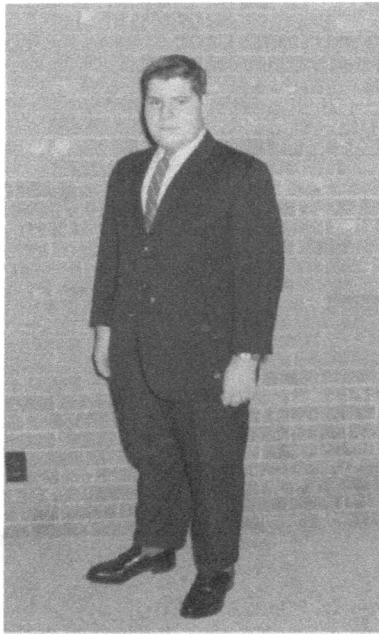

Year 1962, thirteen years old

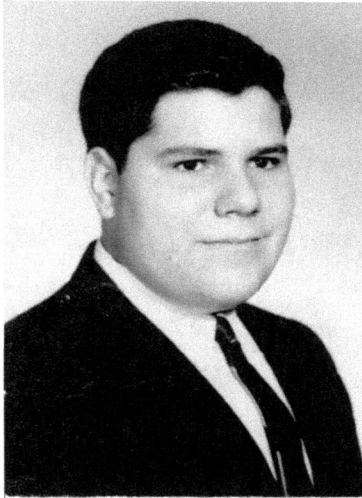

Year 1967, high school graduation,
18 years old

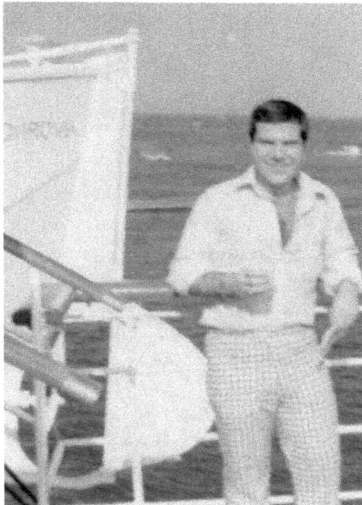

Year 1974 (a handsome devil!),
24 years old, after a year on Weight Watchers ®

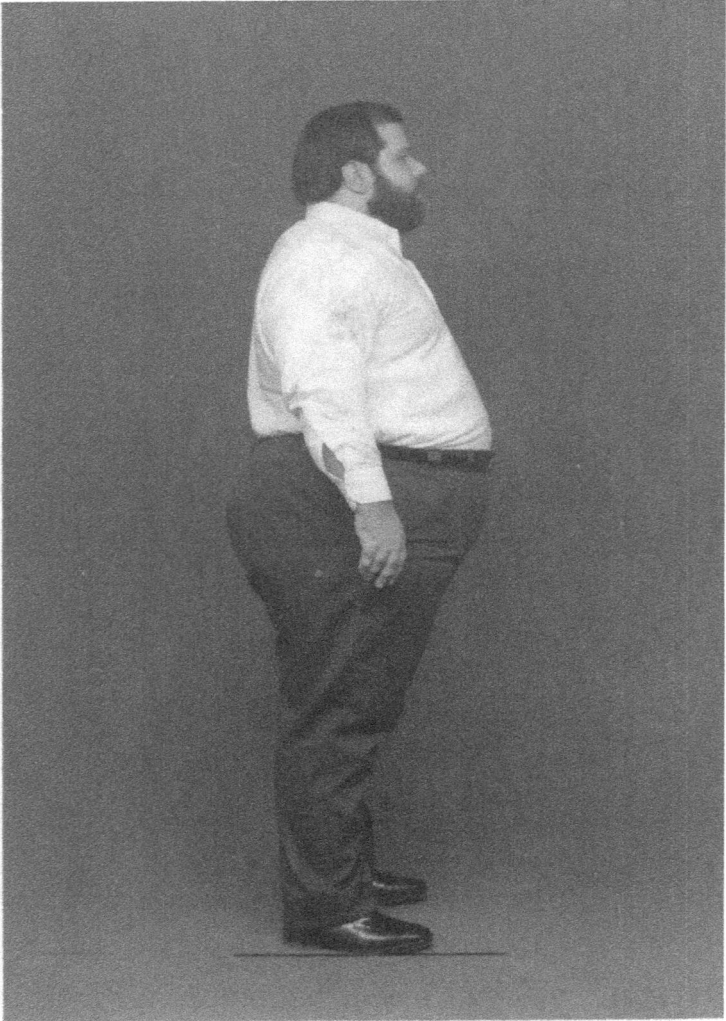

1981, Rice Diet check in photo, 31 years old

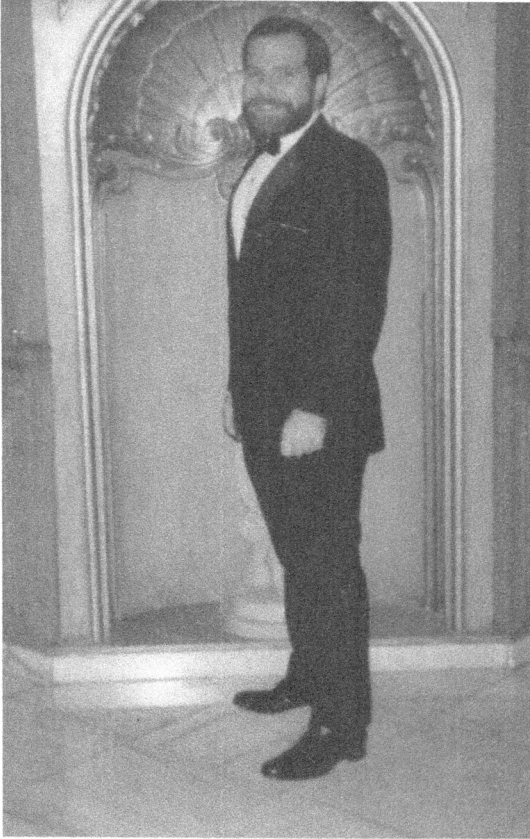

Year 1983, 33 years old
(WOW! - my lowest weight as an adult)

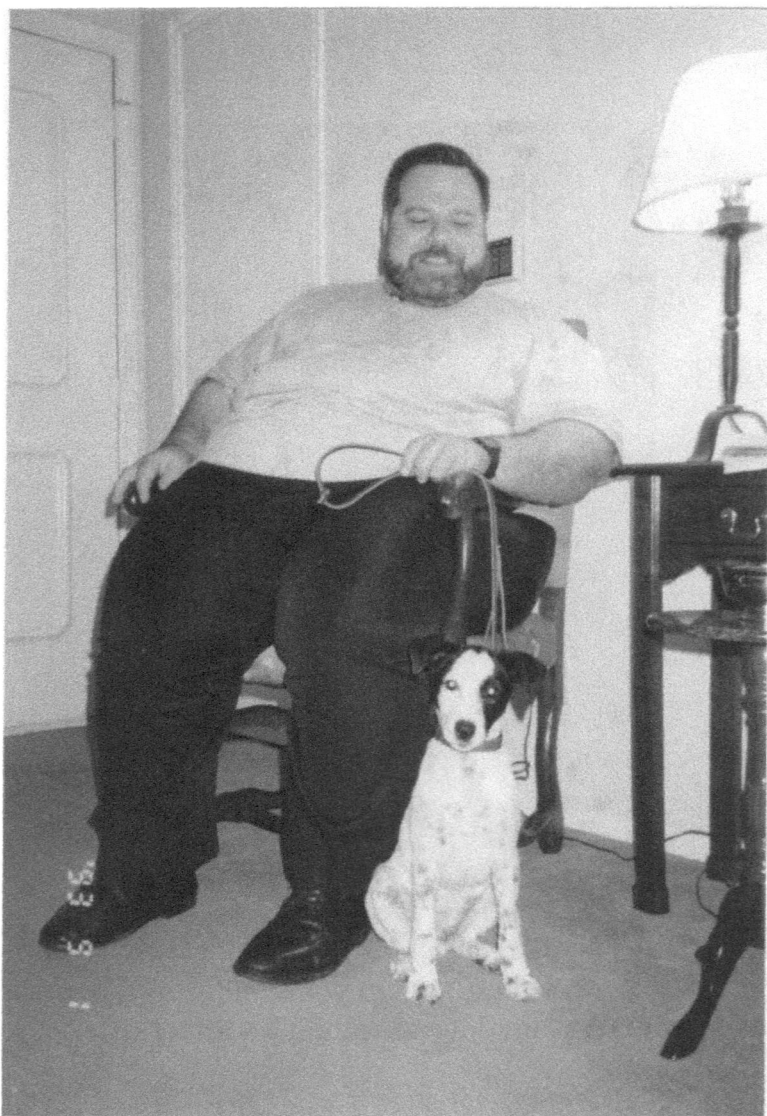

Year 1993, 44 years old
(nearing my highest weight ever!)

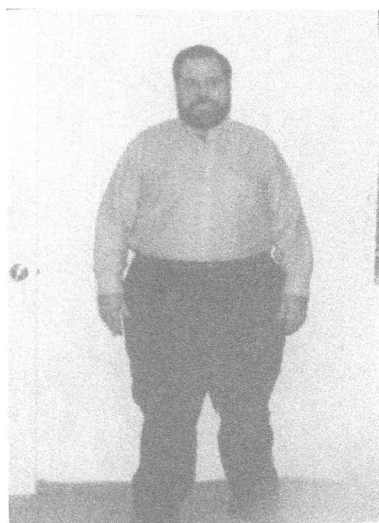

Year 1996 – '97, after using "Phen-fen"

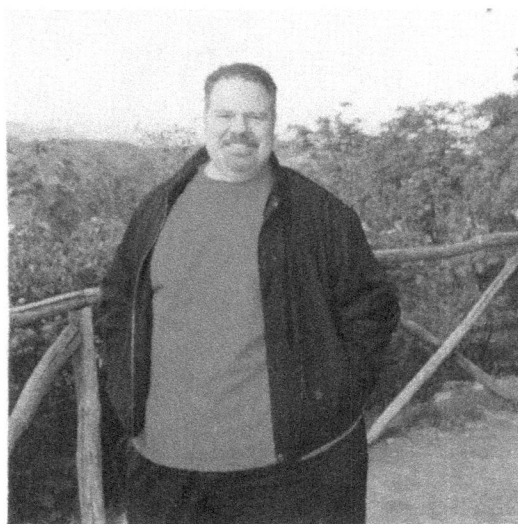

Year 2004, 55 years old (back up again!)

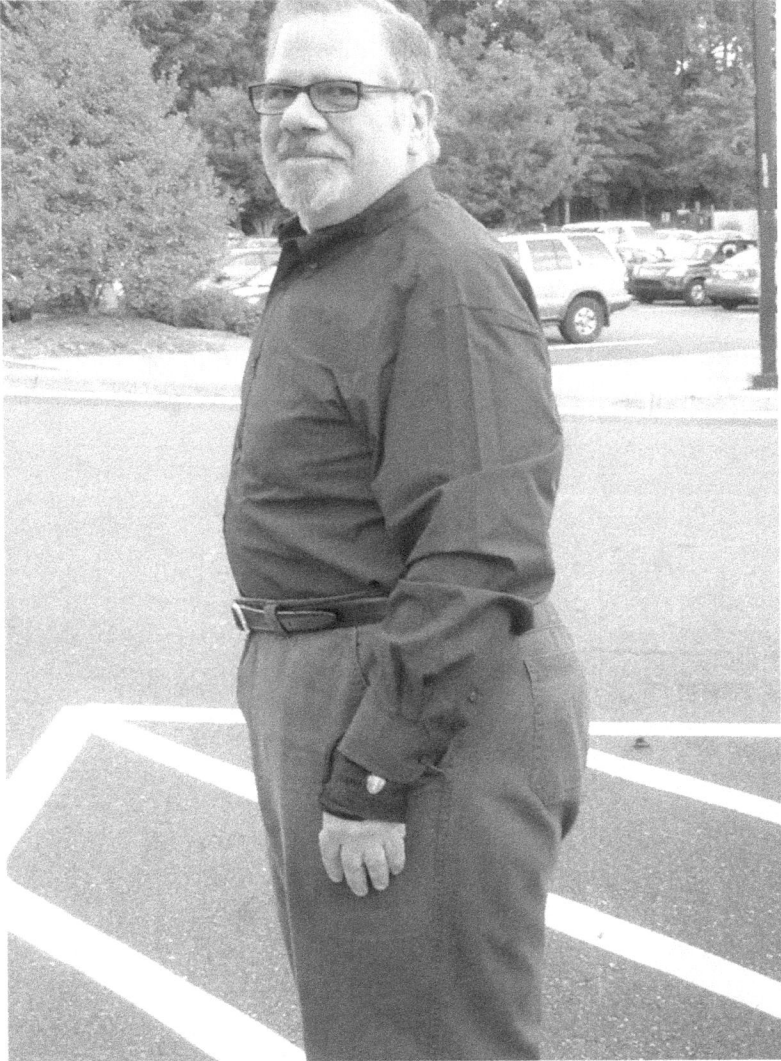

November 2011, 62 years old,
after Rice Diet program
(prior to my cancer diagnosis)

Part Two

Healing

"Our deepest fear is not that we are inadequate. Our deepest fear is that we are powerful beyond measure. It is our light, not our darkness that most frightens us. We ask ourselves, who am I to be brilliant, gorgeous, talented, fabulous? Actually, who are you *not* to be? You are a child of God. Your playing small does not serve the world. There is nothing enlightened about shrinking so that other people won't feel insecure around you. We are all meant to shine, as children do. We were born to make manifest the glory of God that is within us. It's not just in some of us; it's in everyone. And as we let our own light shine, we unconsciously give other people permission to do the same. As we are liberated from our own fear, our presence automatically liberates others."

Quote from - *A Return To Love: Reflections on the Principles of A Course in Miracles©, By Marianne Williamson*

Chapter Five

Introduction — The Healing of the "I"

"The aphorism, 'As a man thinketh in his heart so is he,' not only embraces the whole of a man's being, but is so comprehensive as to reach out to every condition and circumstance of his life. A man is literally what he thinks, his character being the complete sum of all his thoughts." Quote from *As a Man Thinketh* by James Allen

*T*here is a saying, "Nothing changes, if nothing changes!" This statement is so very true. We never-ending dieters keep on the diet roller coaster that takes us up and down, over and over again. We keep riding until we become so tired and weary that we want to get off, but by some superhuman force, we keep riding. As I quoted in a prior chapter, Albert Einstein's saying also strikes a major nerve here: "Insanity: doing the same thing over and over again and expecting different results!"

I knew that there needed to be a major change if I, if we, were going to get off that roller coaster. There needed to be a major shift in how we approach our lives and ourselves. We needed a significant and positive change in our thought processes and beliefs.

When I started to think about what it would take to heal oneself from a history of never-ending dieting, I began an in-depth evaluation of my life as a diet. I took an intense inventory of all the diet attempts that I had made to lose weight. But more important than the diets, I looked at what was happening in my life and what my motivations were for weight loss during these different periods. What had worked? What had not worked?

The most significant self-examination that I did was taking a painstaking look at what types of mental, emotional, physical, and spiritual principles that I was practicing (if any at all) not only during my numerous diet endeavors, but more importantly, in my life. I wanted to determine key human qualities that would help not only me, but also all who have endured dealing with this pink elephant in our lives. These are human qualities that would help motivate us, restructure our thinking, and ultimately heal us from the fat-minded patterns that have kept us in the never-ending diet cycle. This is a process of using these qualities in a way that would lead us to a place of total self-acceptance, unconditional self-love, and just plain being happy! In due course, by being in an unconditional state of acceptance and happiness, the weight loss would follow.

Throughout my dieting history I have met many wonderful people who, like myself, were never-ending dieters, and a number of them have become lifelong friends. Upon completion of the analysis of my diets and my life during these times, I needed to secure some feedback on my conclusions from like-minded dieters. So I shared these hopefully healing qualities that I ascertained from my personal research with some friends to get their input. The responses that I received let me know that I had hit a home run. Now, how did I win the game for me, for all of us never-ending dieters? What process would allow these life changing and life affirming virtues to become second nature to all of us and accelerate our healing process?

After many considerations I came up with a plan and I began to devotedly use this process. This method is not something new, but I geared it toward never-ending dieters like myself and what I know about our minds. I contacted my spiritual mentor, and she helped me to clarify and strengthen my intentions and further develop this plan, this strategy if you will, to help heal me, and to help heal others like myself.

I wanted to utilize my energy with a plan that was effective, yet easy. Though what I am about to share with you is basically quite easy, it does take a consistent, daily commitment to follow through. I found that as soon as I began to practice this method, I began seeing instant results. I am not speaking of weight loss, though I know that has been our ultimate goal. But the goal that I am speaking about here is by far more important than weight loss. Now you are thinking, *What is more important than weight loss?* I understand this thought process all too well and it took me decades to get to this new realization that I am now sharing with you, but the wait was in fact worth it.

I am speaking of a goal of increased self-esteem, true self-love, and letting go of all the crazy obsessions and thought processes that we have when it comes to dieting and our weight. A goal that allows us to achieve a state of well being that permits us to be happier with ourselves and more satisfied in our lives. This is a whole new world for me, and I am sure it will be for you as well.

I must tell you, it feels great and provides a freedom that makes you feel absolutely amazing. It has totally provided me with a major shift in the way I think, feel, and act. It actually quiets and, in some cases, shuts down those awful critical voices that scream at us and won't let us be. It truly helps us to make friends with our individual "Mr. Hyde," and helps to dramatically relieve the obsessions that we have practiced for so many years. I could go on, but this is how the plan works.

THE HEALING PLAN

This plan is simple, easy to use, but will require your daily commitment. Please trust me, it does work. If it can work for me, it will work for you. If you will dedicate yourself and be steadfast with following this action plan, I know that you will begin to feel better.

Perhaps you are skeptical. All I ask is that you put forth one hundred percent of your efforts and give this plan the chance it deserves, the chance you deserve to see a major shift in how you feel, act, and react to life. By mustering your courage and conviction and devoting yourself to this program, you will hopefully unlock and finally live your dreams and aspirations, whatever those may be for you.

This plan is about affirmations, affirmations within the various virtues, the human qualities that I determined need significant shifts in our psyches to lead never-ending dieters to a new way of thinking and acting.

In each of the following chapters on healing, I will briefly discuss each virtue and the shift we need to make into how we think and how we feel within that virtue's meaning. After the discussion, there are affirmations for you to use on a daily basis. I suggest that you focus on each virtue one at a time in the order that I present them, or you can choose one to start with that you feel needs your immediate attention. Your ultimate goal will be to cover all of these qualities in your own time, and at your own pace. What I know is that the quicker you begin the better. The quicker you start the process, the happier you will be and the quicker the healing will occur.

What you need to know about affirmations is that they do work. Affirmations have been a proven method of change for decades. There are documented true stories of people who have healed themselves from major diseases by using affirmations. The brain is an incredible organ and our thought process and beliefs can be changed.

Affirmations are an "I" statement, with an active verb, followed by an affirmative noun that describes who we are, and what we truly know about and for ourselves. An example of an affirmation: "I am fearless and face my world proudly with strength and courage." When you repeat the affirmations, know that they are true and feel their reality for yourself. For some this may seem awkward at first and that critical voice in your head may tell you that what you are affirming is not true. But keep on track and this will change, slower for some, quicker for others.

The affirmations are in a state of being in the NOW! We are not "trying to" do something. "Trying to" is an action of making an effort at something. We want an action of being in the present, now. We are now! What we are affirming is our unconditional state of being in our own truths now, right at this moment, not something that will be in the future. You will be amazed at how quickly you will start to feel happier, healthier, and more satisfied with yourself.

Please remember that the desire to change is paramount in the use of these affirmations. Believe what you say! Know that what you are affirming is, without a doubt, your own personal, present truth.

Let me suggest the following steps to give you a direction in how to use the affirmations:

I.   <u>**WRITE DOWN THE AFFIRMATIONS THAT YOU CHOOSE TO WORK WITH FOR A PARTICULAR VIRTUE**</u>
(Note: At the end of each of the following chapters there are a number of affirmations for your use. You can certainly use all of the affirmations for each virtue, but if this feels too overwhelming for you, choose the two or three that really resonate for you and use those.)

Writing the affirmations down provides a connection from your hand to your brain, and it is a great starting point.

II. **POST YOUR AFFIRMATIONS IN A LOCATION, OR PREFERABLY IN VARIOUS LOCATIONS THAT ARE PRIVATE FOR YOU AND WHERE YOU WILL SEE THEM OFTEN**
Examples: Post them to your bathroom mirror, refrigerator, inside your desk at work, any place where you will see them often. You can also utilize your personal technology by posting the affirmations that you are working on to your cell phone, electronic tablet, and/or on your computer. Whenever you see your affirmations your brain will automatically recognize, repeat, and continue to absorb them. The more locations that you are able to post them, the stronger the message will be to your brain.

III. **DAILY SCHEDULE - REPEAT THE AFFIRMATIONS TO YOURSELF AS OFTEN AS POSSIBLE**
A. **EVERY MORNING WHEN YOU AWAKE, AND BEFORE YOU GET OUT OF BED, SAY THE AFFIRMATIONS TO YOURSELF SILENTLY**
If you live alone, say the affirmations out loud. If you can spare the time, repeat

them two or three times...the more repeated, the better. If you have a hectic household with crazy morning activities, give yourself this one-minute to repeat the affirmations to yourself. Please give yourself this one moment in time as you deserve it so very much.

B. **ONCE OUT OF BED AND IN YOUR BATHROOM, LOOK AT YOURSELF IN THE MIRROR AND AGAIN REPEAT THE AFFIRMATIONS TWO OR THREE TIMES.**
As you look into the mirror, look directly in your eyes, believe and completely know without a doubt that what you are saying is true for you. For some of you, the mirror may be difficult at first, and that is understandable. If it is, find a comfortable place once you are out of bed and repeat the affirmations two or three times, preferably out loud.

(Note: The more you are able to say your affirmations out loud, the greater their power of change for you. Of course there will be times when this is not an option, but the more said out loud, the better!)

C. **DURING THE DAY WHILE DRIVING TO AND FROM WORK, OR RUNNING ERRANDS, REPEAT**

YOUR AFFIRMATIONS TO YOURSELF.

On your coffee breaks or lunch breaks at work, take a minute, take a few deep breaths to relax, and repeat your affirmations. The strategy here is that the more you repeat your affirming statements to yourself, the quicker your brain will start processing and imprinting them as your truth. The quicker and deeper these imprints of truth become, the quicker these positive thoughts will materialize as an integral part of who you are, and your belief in yourself will experience a major change.

D. AT NIGHT BEFORE YOU GO TO SLEEP, ONCE AGAIN, TAKE A MINUTE AND REPEAT YOUR AFFIRMATIONS TO YOURSELF TWO OR THREE TIMES.

Once again, repeating them out loud to yourself while looking in the mirror adds additional strength to the change process.

E. AFTER EACH AFFIRMATION SESSION, GIVE YOURSELF A HUG AND SAY, "AND SO IT IS!"

If you are in a location that will allow you to do this, take your right hand to your left shoulder and your left hand to your right shoulder, and give yourself a long, strong hug, as strong as possible. While you are hugging yourself, say, "And so it is!" This hug is about acknowledging you, congratulating yourself, and loving yourself. We get far too few hugs in our lives and we need to nurture ourselves and give ourselves these loving hugs that we so deserve. It's time! Ultimately, you are letting yourself and the Universe know that whatever affirmations you are saying are true: "And so it is!" This is the ultimate statement of your truth. You are releasing the truth for yourself and who you really are to the entire Universe.

IV.   **RESOLUTION OF YOUR OWN TRUTH –
YOU BELIEVE YOUR AFFIRMATIONS
WITHOUT A DOBUT**

Keep the above process of repeating a set of particular affirmations going for as long as necessary. That "necessary" being until the affirmations you are repeating become second nature to you, and you really believe, you absolutely know without a shadow of a doubt, without reservation, that these statements are one hundred percent true for you. These affirmations are YOU! No doubts, no hesitations; they are all totally true for you. You are now what you say you are! YOUR TRUTH IS NOW TOTALLY INTEGRATED IN YOUR WHOLE BEING!

V.   **MOVING FORWARD TO YOUR NEXT SET OF AFFIRMATIONS**
When you have reached the pinnacle of belief for yourself for a particular virtue, as discussed in IV above, move on to another virtue's set of affirmations. Again, follow the above directions and repeat these new statements until they become the truth of who you really are too. If you wish to continue repeating the previous set(s) of affirmations that you used, that is fine. But if you really have achieved the belief in yourself for a particular set, focus your efforts on the new set. If at any time in your future you feel that there is a slip in your new belief processes, immediately return to the affirmation practice on whatever particular issue that needs to be revisited.

This affirmation process does work. It is easy and the power that we possess within us is amazing. Our ability to change our beliefs in ourselves is ours for the taking. It truly is. "And so it is!"

"It's the repetition of
affirmations that leads to belief.
And once that belief becomes deep conviction,
things begin to happen." - Muhammad Ali

Let the healing begin...

Chapter Six

On Being Brave

"What's the bravest thing you ever did?...
Getting up this morning, he said."
- Cormac McCarthy, *The Road*

I felt that our healing journey needed to begin with the realization of who we really are--very brave individuals! The one thing I know about all of us never-ending dieters is that we are brave. It is difficult being fat. It is hard to constantly fight the universe with what we feel is a battle that we cannot seem to win no matter what we do.

But what I unequivocally know is that WE ARE BRAVE! Whether you are twenty pounds or two hundred pounds overweight, it is a battle for us physically, mentally, emotionally, and spiritually. But somehow, someway, we dig deep down into our beings and we find the strength and courage to move on, minute after minute, day after day, week after week, and year after year. We may feel like giving up at times, but the truth is that we never give up. Never! We seem to follow the old adage that if at first you don't succeed, try and try again!

We tend to think of ourselves as weak, as failures, but the truth is that as a group we are probably some of the strongest and most dedicated individuals in the world. We are from all walks of life. We are women, men, teens, and even children. We are from all professions, all races, all religions, of all ages, from different countries, and the one thing that we have in common is that we all want to lose weight to be healthy, to finally win this crazy battle that we have been fighting for many years, and for some, our entire lives.

Again, the good news is that we are not alone. We are all out there, and now is the time that we come together. The brave, meet the brave!

I know who you are. You are a survivor. You are someone who travels down one path, and if this path does not take you to your destination, you try another. You keep going no matter what. It is unfortunate that you do not realize this about yourself, but I do. I know who you are, and like me, you keep on trying.

Brave is a strong word and that is exactly who you are. You are a brave, courageous, outstanding individual who has survived a hard road and you keep on truckin'! You may get sidetracked and travel aimlessly for a while, but you always find your way back. Then, when you do find your way back, you accelerate and advance onward to new heights.

Do we get diverted and lost at times? Yes, of course. Life happens and we get redirected and unfocused for whatever reason. We would not be human if we didn't. Do we stay there and wallow in our pity? Sometimes, yes, we do. But ultimately, we pick ourselves up, dust ourselves off, and start over.

If you are like me you feel as though you have failed, and more specifically that you are a failure with your diet history. But you are not a failure. Not at all. It takes brave individuals to pick themselves up and move forward again. We do just that, and congratulations for doing it.

You know, life is hard. We have a lot of balls to juggle on a daily basis. First, we have ourselves to take care of. If you have a family, you have your significant other and/or children to be there for and take care of as well. Then there are the bills, the bosses, the house and car repairs, our health issues and the health issues of our loved ones, ad infinitum. On top of it all, you deal with your weight and dieting. It takes a powerful person to handle and deal with all of these responsibilities, and you do it, and you do it well. Please, know that you are an incredibly strong individual and you deserve to believe in yourself and your powers. You deserve to know that you are brave! In fact, in my opinion, we are the bravest of the brave.

These affirmations are about affirming who you really are, finally realizing who you are, and living in this truth. In addition to accepting ourselves without hesitation, doubt, or reservation, I want you to know that you are brave. I want you to believe that you are brave, a remarkable survivor, and intuitively know that you will accomplish anything that you set out to do. You are brave!

Please remember the desire to change is paramount in the use of these affirmations. Practice these daily and often (preferably repeated out loud), and you will start to see changes in how you feel sooner than you think. The main thing is that you give yourself the chance you deserve to see the change. Remember, you are worthy! You are the best and deserve the best! You are brave!

AFFIRMATIONS ON BEING BRAVE

1) I proudly realize and accept that I am brave and act with confidence.

2) I am fearless and face my world proudly with strength and courage.

3) I continually prove that I am brave and totally support this truth for myself.

4) I am filled with confidence and it shows to the world.

5) I am brave!

AND SO IT IS!

(Now, give yourself that big hug!)

NOTE: As you begin to master the thoughts of these affirmations, please read the next chapter on "Acceptance." The affirmations on acceptance work well together with those presented above.

Chapter Seven

Acceptance

"You yourself, as much as anybody in the entire
universe, deserve your love and affection."
– Gautama Buddha

I talk with my best friend Tom on a daily basis. Tom
is one of the few people in my life with whom I can
say or do anything, and he loves and accepts me for
me, no matter what. There are no secrets between us.
Tom is a very wise man and also understands the
emotions and mentality of never-ending dieters
because he has experienced periods of perpetual
dieting in his own life. Tom is my personal captive
audience and I could, and would, complain about my
weight, my failed efforts, and the effects that these
had on me in all areas of my life. He would listen and
commiserate with me. My complaining to him
happened on a regular basis, and often multiple times
within a day.

After going through a metamorphosis regarding his
own weight and dieting, Tom had a major shift in how
he thought of himself and his related weight and diet
issues. So one morning, as I was doing my usual
complaining about being fat, Tom said to me, "What

we resist persists! If you keep complaining about being fat and not being happy with yourself, you will continue to stay that way. Love and accept yourself just the way you are, at this very moment, right now! You are an incredibly wonderful man just the way you are, fat and all. You let your fat define you and that is not who Maurice truly is! When you have mastered self-love and total acceptance of yourself, fat and all, every minute of every day, deep within every cell of your being, then the changes you want to make in your life will begin to happen, including losing your weight."

Tom's (for want of a better word) confrontation was a wake-up call. In my heart I knew what Tom said to me was true. Yet at the same time, it was completely foreign to me because my life had been about being fat, dieting, and treating myself in the resulting manner to which I had become accustomed, thus complaining accordingly. I was in a state of unhappiness and self-loathing because I persisted in thinking and acting the same way that I had been for decades.

I analyzed Tom's words to me, thought about them on a very deep, emotional level, and they are so true. "What we resist persists!" If we continue to live with these negative thoughts that are constantly generating damaging messages to us, and in turn, these harmful messages result in our continuing to live and react to life as we do, then we will continue to believe and treat ourselves in a negative, self-defeating manner. We will continue to believe that because we are fat (whatever fat means to you individually), we are not worthy, not pretty, not deserving, or not whatever it is that is negative to you personally. We will continue to procrastinate making a change because what we have become to believe about ourselves persists and is actually a false sense of being that has become a comfortable reality for us. Ultimately, by resisting change we stay in our current state of unhappiness.

At some point in our lives our self-esteem began deteriorating. Much of what we believe about ourselves is formatted in our brains from our early childhood. Additionally, certain life events, crisis, and/or situations can also affect our self-esteem negatively.

For me, my poor self-image started in early childhood with being a fat kid and having to endure the constant harassment from my school peers. My family led me to believe that there was something wrong with me because I was fat, that I was different from others, and that I needed help. The development of my poor self-esteem started very early and continued with my life as a diet.

For others, it happens during the different phases in their lives. Maybe it was being teased and called "fatty" in junior high and high school. Maybe we were not invited to a social event or dance and just knew it was because of our weight. We have seen in today's news what the bullying of peers within our schools lead to. Yet years ago we endured such hurtful bullying and it destroyed our self-esteem.

A woman has a family and keeps on some of her pregnancy weight with each child. With time, her weight accelerates and her self-esteem begins to crumble. Or the athletic man who was a real jock during his high school and college days; he gets married, has a family, works a sedentary desk job, the pounds come on, and with time his self-esteem deteriorates.

Then of course there is the commercial fashion industry that has shown us ultrathin models for decades, creating a false vision of what everyday people should look like, male as well as female. These images were present in all forms of media and we were constantly bombarded with these images beginning in our 'tween years. If we allowed these fashion model bodies to become the goal for our own bodies, this began a path to our self-destructive thinking ultimately leading us to the creation of being another never-ending dieter, or worse, to someone who developed a severe eating disorder in trying to achieve an unrealistic fashion model body.

Whatever the situation, whatever happened to us in our individual histories that made us believe we are not worthy, that we are underserving people because of our weight, it is just not true! I will say this with great conviction and love, that some of the kindest, most intelligent, creative, interesting, and just plain good people whom I have ever met in my life are never-ending dieters. I know you are one of those magnificent people too!

We have been beaten down, hurt, ostracized, discriminated against, called names, and we cried too many tears over our weight issues and what we believe to have been "failures" of all of our diet attempts. The beliefs and imprints that we have created in our brains are not who we really are. We are not the negative labels that our critical voice tells us we are. Our real truth is that we are wonderful, loving, intelligent, fun, exciting individuals who are courageous fighters. Not only are we fighters, but we are super survivors.

The thing about poor self-esteem is that it keeps us stuck. It is not the diets, it is not the fat, but our thought processes that are keeping us stuck. The willingness to allow change to happen is scary. The unknown is scary, but the outcomes of change are amazing. Developing a new outlook for yourself by going from the negative beliefs that you have existed with to the new positives of the real you, will open new windows of opportunity and make your life shine and dazzle like it has never before. You will see a difference not only in yourself, but also in reactions to you from your families, friends, work colleagues, and an all around change for the better in all areas of your lives. Every day will be an adventure and we will not be stuck in a negative cycle that our weighted mind has kept us in. Doesn't this sound exciting and wonderful? It can be yours, now! Embrace who you really are, and you are going to be amazed at what happens.

Please remember the desire to change is paramount in the use of these affirmations. Practice these daily and often, and you will start to see changes in how you feel sooner than you think. The main thing is to give yourself the chance you deserve to see the change. Remember, you are worthy! You are magnificent! You are your own miracle!

AFFIRMATIONS ON ACCEPTANCE

1) I love myself unconditionally and accept myself just as I am right now.

2) I approve of myself in every way and it makes me feel great.

3) Every day, and in every way, I am thankful for who I am in body, mind, and soul.

4) I lovingly reclaim myself by accepting all parts of me.

5) I unconditionally love, accept, and respect myself for the wonderful man/woman that I am.

6) I love and accept myself past, present, and future.

AND SO IT IS!
(ALWAYS REMEMBER
TO HUG YOURSELF, ALWAYS!)

Chapter Eight

Forgiveness

"To forgive is the highest, most beautiful form of love.
In return, you will receive untold
peace and happiness."
- Robert Muller

When I look at my life as a diet, I realize that I have a tendency to judge myself solely on my past diet endeavors. I look back and think, *What if I had done that differently? What if this had happened?* or *What if that had occurred?* The "what-if," the "should have," the "could have," and the "why didn't I?" play over and over in my mind. I get so involved in all of the mind gibberish of analyzing my past that I lose sight of this very moment and what is happening to me now. Regrets and our constant rehashing of the past do one thing: they keep us chained to our pasts.

Forgiveness goes hand and hand with self-love and self-acceptance as discussed in the previous chapter. As I have stated, we are courageous fighters. The unfortunate part of our fights is that each of us, individually, are our own greatest opponent.

If you are a parent, how many times have you forgiven your children for the wrongs they have done?

When you think back on your own parents and how they brought you up, you forgive them for their wrongdoings and let go of their mistakes because you realize, I hope, that they were doing the best they could with the skills they had. If you are, or have ever been pet owners, need I even approach the numerous times that we have forgiven our four-legged children for their mischief or the accidents that were out of their control? We do forgive, constantly, and we love unconditionally through our forgiveness.

But the one person, the most important person, in our lives that we need to forgive is ourselves. How much longer do we need to relive the past and all the diets we have been on? How much longer do we have to feel so awful about ourselves because of our weight? How much longer are we going to let our thoughts and our critical voice hold us back from participating in life fully?

Enough is enough! We have hurt and allowed ourselves to exist in a wounded state of being long enough. We have every right to feel good and be happy like every other human walking this earth. It is our birthright to be happy and healthy, not to be sad, angry, anxious, or depressed and living in the past. Now is now and the past is the past. Now is the time! Now is YOUR time!

If we are truly thorough about forgiving ourselves, letting go of the past, and loving ourselves unconditionally, we will see a dramatic change not only in our lives but also in all those around us, including our relationships. In addition, if we can really dig deep and forgive all of the people and/or situations from our pasts who have hurt us and keeps us harboring anger or regret, we will totally cleanse ourselves for a new beginning to our lives.

Through forgiveness we will no longer abuse ourselves with food or self-deprecation. We will experience joy and excitement with each new day. We will welcome waking up, getting out of bed, and be thankful for another day to be alive and enjoy the world rather than lying there and thinking of all the excuses to stay in bed and hibernate from life.

Through my own experience with the affirmation practice on my own self-acceptance and forgiveness, I feel a newfound peace and love for myself like I have never felt before. Forgiveness is so freeing and it releases us from the chains of our pasts that have been holding us back, not only in our weight loss efforts but in everything we do.

I would also like to include a special message here to those of you who have had the unfortunate involvement of experiencing a traumatic event or period in your life that may be one of the causes of your staying in your never-ending diet cycles. My first hope is that you have sought the professional help that you need and have come to terms with acceptance and forgiveness for whatever your event(s) was, as well as the participants in that event. If you have not sought professional help, please seek it out now. Not coming to terms with your past traumatic event(s) and not letting go of the stigmas related to these memories will only support your continued suffering, hold you back from being the person you are truly meant to be, and keep you from enjoying the joyful life that you deserve.

My wish for you all is that you are willing to do the affirmation work necessary to forgive yourself. You really do have this power. If you do the affirmations daily, are patient and give the affirmations the time necessary to alter your thought processes, you will experience a major change and shift in your being. You will experience a magnificent release and a new freedom like the one that I am personally experiencing in my life from my affirmation practice on forgiveness.

Below there are eight affirmations. The last two affirmations allow you to personally select a person and/or situations specific to yourself that you wish to forgive. Select the affirmations that mean the most to you for your affirmation practice and you can always adjust your usage of these if you feel the necessity to do so. Again, I would like to emphasize that repeating your affirmations out loud and as often as possible gives them a greater impact for your healing.

Please remember the desire to change is paramount in the use of these affirmations. The power is within you! Know that what you are affirming for yourself is your truth, without any doubts or hesitations.

You deserve to love yourself! You deserve to let go of the past and live for the now! Forgive yourself, others, and a whole new world will open for you.

AFFIRMATIONS ON FORGIVENESS

(Note: the number 6 affirmation below has been included for those who have experienced a traumatic event in their lives)

1) I totally forgive myself for the mistakes that I believed I have made and set myself free from the past.

2) I happily release the past and I am at peace.

3) I willingly let go of the past. The past no longer has any power over me and I move forward with ease.

4) I set myself free from all anger, resentment, guilt, and self-loathing and move into the future with total acceptance.

5) The past is past and I am living joyfully in the present moment.

6) I now release all past traumas and caringly embrace myself with love.

FOR SPECIFIC FORGIVENESS YOU WISH TO GIVE:

7) I lovingly forgive myself for <u>(put whatever you need to forgive yourself for here)</u>.

8) I let go of the past and forgive <u>(name of person or persons)</u> and move forward with total freedom.

"Make peace with the past so it won't screw up the present." – Regina Brett

AND SO IT IS!

(Hug yourself...one more time...
and again, one more time!)

Chapter Nine

Gratitude

"Acknowledging the good that you already have in
your life is the foundation for all abundance."
– Eckhart Tolle,
A New Earth: Awakening to Your Life's Purpose

*D*o you ever feel like you are different from
everyone else in the world? At times, do you feel
sorry for yourself from this thought process of being
different, leading you deeper into stages of self-hatred
and unhappiness? Do you feel that because you are
overweight that you are a victim and that you have to
constantly compensate for who you are as a person? If
you have any of these specific or related thoughts or
feelings, I understand you totally.

Have you ever taken the time to look and really see
what is going on with people in the world around us?
Do you ever see a young child in a wheelchair,
knowing that this child has a disease that does not
allow him or her to walk, or worse? Have you ever seen
a paraplegic or quadriplegic maneuvering themselves
in and out of cars, wheelchairs, or both? Have you seen
any bald individuals and it quickly becomes clear to
you that they have obviously lost their hair due to

chemotherapy in their battle with cancer? The world of those "less fortunate" than we are is all around us. At least, this is how we see these individuals and have empathy for them.

But I would be willing to bet you that ninety-nine percent of these individuals whom you see and believe to be "unfortunate" within their situations are actually happy and dealing with their personal obstacles quite comfortably.

I understand fully that we all have our problems and many of us consider our being overweight to be the major one in our life. We wake up with our weight and diet concerns, and go to sleep with them. But so does the person with multiple sclerosis, the person battling cancer, and the quadriplegic. They too wake up and go to sleep with their dire situations. Our plight is very real to us and it should be. But we cannot allow it to rule us.

It's time that we look at our glass as half full and not half empty. The truth that we are the lucky ones. Yes, we are fat. Yes, we have to work at losing our excess weight. But unless we have something else monumental to deal with, we are lucky just to be fat. This really is our truth if we think about what other conditions we might have to be dealing with in our lives.

We tend to forget how lucky we truly are and to be grateful for what we have in our lives. The concept of gratitude has been around since the dawn of man. We see it in our religions. We see it in our therapies. We see it all over the media in our talk shows. One of the biggest advocates of gratitude is Oprah Winfrey.

Oprah brought "being grateful" to the forefront of society through her talk show and magazine, helping to change and enrich the lives of many people.

The fact is that being grateful works. For myself, I know that when I started to take the time to verbally express my gratitude for all that I am thankful for, no matter how small or great, as well as actually writing a gratitude list, it made a world of difference in how I feel, and more importantly how I see the world and live my daily life. I am grateful for everything. I am grateful for waking up in the morning and being given the opportunity to be alive and live for another day. I am grateful for my family, for my friends, for the clothes on my back, for the food on my table, and for the money in my checking account. By being grateful for it all, small and great, my life changed. I am happier, healthier, and more satisfied in my entire life.

One of the main things that I want all us to be grateful for is our bodies. Being overweight takes a big toll on us over the years. Whether you have been overweight since childhood or you became overweight in your adult years, excess weight stresses our bodies.

But our bodies are amazing machines. Our bodies have seen us through a lot of abuse and difficult challenges. I know full well of these difficulties and challenges as I shared with you in the chapter on "Me and the Big C." One thing I have become very grateful for is my body, and it is very important for you to be grateful for your body as well. Our bodies have carried us through sickness and health. We have all had our aches and pains, ills, surgeries, health crises, and the like. But we are still here. There is a Stephen

Sondheim song with lyrics that express it so well: "Good times and bum times, I've seen them all, and, my dear, I'm still here!"

We are here and we need to say "Thank you, body! Thank you for continuing to work no matter how much I put you through." Our bodies are miracles. Your body is a miracle!

The affirmations below that I developed and use have helped me in becoming a happier and healthy person, and much more satisfied with my life. The specific affirmations are followed by one that you can fill in with something specific that you are individually grateful for. Let yourself relax and just go for it. Be grateful for every little thing that you have.

Please remember the desire to change is paramount in the use of these affirmations. Your body is a miracle! Your life is a miracle! You are a miracle!

AFFIRMATIONS ON GRATITUDE

1) I am grateful for everything that I have in my life at this very moment.

2) I am genuinely thankful for being alive today and for all of my life-enriching experiences.

3) My body is amazing and I am so very grateful for how it carries me through life so powerfully.

4)   I am thankful for my good health and
abundant life.

5)   I am sincerely grateful for (fill in what you
are personally grateful for here). (Note: If
you really want express results, begin
writing a daily gratitude list of ALL things
you are grateful for by using this
affirmation to help you make your list...it
works!)

AND SO IT IS!

(REMEMBER TO GIVE YOURSELF THAT BIG HUG!)

Chapter Ten

Health

"The greatest wealth is health." – Virgil

Without a doubt, health is the most important issue for the healing of never-ending dieters. A majority of us already know the truth about how being overweight negatively affects our health, but it is worth repeating again and again. For all of us, good health, being happy, and to live long lives are our primary goals.

For the younger readers, your goals are more likely focused on looking better, sex appeal, and great clothes. Ah sweet youth! These are understandable goals for you. But ultimately, it is very important to educate yourself now about the benefits of better health. It is about loving ourselves enough to come to terms with the fact that what we are dealing with is truly a life-and-death issue.

We keep moving through life day after day, year after year being overweight with our continued never-ending diet attempts. Overtime, being overweight can and usually does cause damage to our bodies and to our health. It is a proven fact that being overweight shortens our life spans. Excess weight affects our joints and mobility. It is a known fact that being overweight is a one of the major causes in the development of diabetes. Being overweight dramatically increases the chance of cardiac and pulmonary issues, elevated blood pressure, and increased incidents of heart attacks and strokes. Being fat is also a major contributing factor for developing cancer, which I discovered the hard way. You know, I love to be positive and keep things light, but this topic is the one that I really want to hit home.

The medical community has stated that in the long run, instead of constant yo-yo (never-ending) dieting it is better to maintain weight at a higher level than putting our bodies through the constant stress of dieting, subsequent weight gains, and then more dieting. BUT, the fact remains that keeping excess weight on our bodies eventually beats them down and affects our longevity over time.

It has been shown that being as little as ten percent over what is considered a normal body weight can have adverse affects on one's health over the years. Not only does the excess weight affect our organs, but our skeletal system breaks down as well. Having personally dealt with obesity and never-ending dieting my entire life ultimately broke down my knees to the point of requiring me to have knee replacements. This is a frequent occurrence for overweight individuals. It's no fun and takes a huge bite out of life. Being overweight not only severely affected my mobility, but also affected me in many other areas of my health including having high blood pressure, the respiratory issue of sleep apnea, the psychological affects of anxiety and depression, and of course cancer with obesity being my only risk factor. It is hard to face reality at times, but obesity is a destructive force on our health.

I know that many of you are shaking your heads and saying to yourselves, "I know all this." But I think at times many of us lose sight of the big picture allowing our focus to drift back to looking better and wanting to get to a certain weight by a specific date or for an upcoming special occasion. The big picture, the main goal dear friends, is without a doubt health, health, health!

One more comment on this issue. If you are like me, you hate when you need to go to the doctor. You know that the "monster scale" is waiting for you and the doctor will tell you, yet once again, that you must lose weight. But please do not let that stop you from going to get regular checkups. Something may be going on that requires medical attention.

Okay, my sermon is over. But I hope you know that this is included with heartfelt concern, and the hope that you will always remember that health is our number one priority in our weight loss endeavors.

Please remember the desire to change is paramount in the use of these affirmations. Below is an extended list of affirmations on health. Using all of them would be ideal. But if you feel that there are too many for you to use, please select the three or four that really resonate for you. You deserve to be healthy! You deserve to be happy! You deserve to live a long, exciting life!

AFFIRMATIONS FOR GOOD HEALTH

1) Being healthy is my birthright and I claim it now.

2) Every cell in my body emits high energy and radiates good health.

3) I lovingly embrace my body, mind, and soul, and as a result, I glow with good health.

4) I maintain good health by taking care of myself by eating healthfully, staying active, and getting a good night's sleep.

5) I am stress free, I stay calm under pressure, and I do not sweat the small stuff in life.

6) I enjoy perfect health by continually making the right choices for my body.

7) I consciously choose to properly nourish my healthy body.

AND SO IT IS!

(HUG TIME!)

Chapter Eleven

On Being Perfect

"But I am learning that perfection isn't what matters.
In fact, it's the very thing that can
destroy you if you let it."
- Emily Giffin, *Something Borrowed*

*I*f you are like me, you want to do to things
perfectly. But the truth is, what is perfect? Perfect
is something that we each define in our own way. For
most of us, perfect is a strict, by-the-book, no-
diversions, all-or-nothing rule that we have lived by
and practiced.

When we write something in long hand, we make
sure that the grammar is perfect, that every "i" is
dotted and every "t" is properly crossed. In our
business lives we make sure that we do everything not
merely first class, but the ultimate, absolute best,
beyond first class.

In our personal lives, we go to great efforts to make
sure that we look perfect. We may not like the
reflections that we see in the mirror, but we make sure
that every hair is in place, the makeup is perfect, and
we look at what we think is perfect in that moment.

As never-ending dieters we are definitely perfectionists. I have worked on trying to ease up on my perfectionism practices many times in the past, but I have yet to master it. This time, let's do it together and finally get it right!

Whenever we go on a diet we get our momentum revved up to maximum intensity. We move quickly and efficiently in being successful at following our diet program and doing what needs to be done. We make sure that we have the proper foods on hand, we have read the diet instructions numerous times to make sure that we understand it, and we have looked at a calendar to determine how much weight we plan to lose by a certain date or event. If we are really dedicated we will actually exercise too. Now that's a "WOW!"

So what is it about perfectionism in dieting that makes us stop moving forward? For me, it is that one bite. If I am following a diet program and deviate with just one bite, all effort stops and any progress that I have made is ignored. My mind tells me that I am a failure and that I haven't done it exactly the way I am supposed to. I have not done it perfectly.

So whether it is a single bite, a meal that deviates from the program, or an all-out binge, the party's over! It's over and I am headed down the road of no return quickly to my old habits. There is a saying that old habits die hard, and it is so true. We can be on a program for months, and one deviation can send us packing right back to our old destructive habits that we have been practicing for so long in our pasts.

This is a hard one and a huge stumbling block for many of us. But we can come to terms with it and really work on changing our perfectionistic practices.

The main thing to come to terms with is that there really is no perfect. We need to realize that the one bite, that one meal, that one binge does not undo weeks, or months, or even years of our efforts. We need to realize that if we do have a slip in our diet, it is just that, a slip. This one action or episode does not change what we have been doing and we need to realize and accept it as okay no matter what. But the most important thing we need to do is to forgive ourselves at that very moment and not let the slip send us into a relapse of nonstop eating. Forgive ourselves immediately, it is now in the past, and we are again moving in a positive, forward direction. Okay, I had that taste, that one bite. I ate that celebratory birthday dinner and indulged. Okay, I used food to soothe me from the hurt that I was dealing with in this situation or that event I had to go to. But these episodes do not undo our efforts to date. We need to say, "STOP! Hold on!" We need to hug ourselves and realize that we are a success. We are doing great and we have made it to this point in time, and we need to congratulate ourselves, not beat ourselves up.

The actual fact, the real truth, is that we are perfect. We are perfect at this very moment. At this point in time, we are pure perfection. This perfection is not changed by a bite, a meal, or a binge that we may partake of that is off our diet programs. With every imperfection that we feel we may have, we are absolutely perfect just the way we are. No matter how loud our critical voice becomes, telling us how bad we are because we "went off" our diet, or how the judgment committee in our head tells us that we are not good enough, not worthy, look awful, and calls us disgusting, it is just not true! We are perfect at this very moment. We are perfect, period! Let us not let that one bite, meal, or binge determine who we are, or our future efforts.

Please remember the desire to change is paramount in the use of these affirmations. You are worthy! You are wonderful! You are perfect just the way you are, no matter what actions that you take in your life! You are perfection!

AFFIRMATIONS TO RELEASE PERFECTIONISM

1) I am my own best friend and treat myself with compassion and understanding.

2) I am free to make mistakes without judgment, knowing that nothing can interfere with my plans and ultimate goals.

3) I unconditionally accept all of my actions as a learning experience and continue to move toward my goal no matter what.

4) I trust in the process of life and know that my good is unfolding with perfect timing.

5) I am relaxed and focused as I follow my plan of action.

6) I choose this moment as a new beginning for growth and peace.

7) I speak to myself respectfully and lovingly in all situations and in all actions that I take.

AND SO IT IS!

(TIME FOR THAT BIG SELF-HUG, OR TWO!)

Chapter Twelve

Stuck in the Middle with You

"Don't walk behind me; I may not lead. Don't walk in
front of me; I may not follow. Just walk
beside me and be my friend."
– Albert Camus

On one occasion when I was in therapy, I discussed
"Mr. Hyde," my critical voices, and how they each
affected me and my weight loss efforts. I told the
therapist how Mr. Hyde would take control of my
actions in an instant and quickly lead me down the
path of self-destruction with food. Additionally, I told
her how those critical voices, that judgment committee
in my psyche would say very negative and hurtful
statements about me. Statements like, "You are fat
and disgusting," or "You should be ashamed of
yourself," leading me to even more self-destructive
behaviors, at times isolation, and the worst of all, self-
hate. I believe that most of you will relate.

After discussing these parts of my behavioral mind,
the therapist said something that really hit me hard.
The therapist said, "Have you ever thought about

making friends with these different parts of you? Obviously they are an integral part of who you are. You have a lifelong history with these parts and they will probably never go away. If you befriend them, perhaps your resulting behaviors will not be as destructive, and maybe you will even have a major shift in how you react to the critical voice judgments and Mr. Hyde's control."

I thought about the therapist's suggestion for days and realized it to be true. We all have parts of ourselves that we do not like. We all have parts of our psyche that we want to change. What if we did befriend those parts of us that have been so self-destructive? Maybe my making friends with these self-destructive parts, they would become less active. Maybe by making peace with them, we could actually control our behaviors.

So how do we make friends with these parts? We start by exercising our own power, our own control, by consciously recognizing these parts and acknowledging their existence both in and out of the time frames of their control and negative declarations. I began practicing this recognition exercise consistently. I developed and practiced affirmations to make peace with and befriend these parts of my mind. Very quickly the intensity of Mr. Hyde's behavior control became much less active in leading me to food to ease my pains and comfort my fears. When the critical voices would start their self-talk and negative statements, I would stop, listen, and let them know that what they were saying about me was not true, that I appreciated their input, but that they needed to know that my real truth was, in fact, the opposite of what they were screaming at me. After my continued practice with the affirmations and recognizing all these parts of me, the voices may still come up at times, and Mr. Hyde may still attempt to control me, but our relationship has changed dramatically.

We all have our own "Mr. Hyde," our own metaphors for our personal fears, demons, or whatever you wish to call them. We definitely all have those critical voices or judgment committees in our heads that unfairly judge us and send us those horrid, negative messages. If we start acknowledging the voice(s) and let them know that we will not accept their judgments as truths, and then steadfastly tell them what our real self-truths are, the less active they will become and we will experience greater peace within ourselves.

Again, this takes time, but it does work. The more you practice, the quicker the results. I hope that these affirmations help you to make peace with those parts of your psyche that have been negative influences and led you to self-destructive thinking and behaviors. Ultimately, we cannot make them disappear, but we can see a drastic reduction in their activity and the power that we have allowed them to exercise over us. By making peace with these destructive parts of ourselves, we will see an increase in our self-esteem and our ability to achieve our goals, whether those are weight loss or other desired victories.

Please remember the desire to change is paramount in the use of these affirmations. You have the power to control your destiny! You are one whole being with all parts working together in perfect harmony!

AFFIRMATIONS ON BEFRIENDING OUR MINDS' PARTS

1) I acknowledge my critical voices and let them know the real truth of my own perfection.

2) I am one whole being with all parts working together in perfect harmony for my highest good.

3) I effectively replace all fears and negative judgments of myself with love, positive thoughts, and self-respect.

4) I maintain a positive course of action and I am successful in all areas of my life.

5) I take control over my thoughts and actions, allowing me to powerfully achieve my goals.

AND SO IT IS!

(HUG YOURSELF...NOW HUG YOURSELF AGAIN!)

Chapter Thirteen

Crisis Hotline

"That which does not kill us makes us stronger."
– Nietzsche

So the auto repair man says, "Your repairs are going to run you about $1,500." And you are already struggling to make ends meet. Next, your boss tells you, "Sorry, but we are going to need you to work overtime for the next three weeks and we cannot let you take the time off that you had previously requested." The doctor looks at you intensely and says, "I am sorry to tell you that you have a cancerous tumor in your right kidney until proven otherwise.You need surgery as soon as possible!"

Life happens! Unfortunately, a part of life is being informed of very unpleasant, sometimes traumatizing news like the examples above. Many of the occurrences that burst into our lives so unexpectedly turn out to be a crisis, particularly those dealing with health, family, work, and/or finances. As a never-ending dieter, and if you are like me, when these crises arise you turn to the one thing that will give you temporary peace, an instant gratification, an immediate escape, and soothe your anxiety and fears. That one thing is food.

We are creatures of habit, and if not habit, our Mr. Hyde surfaces and takes over for us. It is the fight or flight syndrome. With the fight, the crisis hits, we stand tall, cry our tears, make a plan, and move forward to deal with it. With flight, we let our Mr. Hyde take control and end up at the cookies aisle in the grocery store or in the fast-food drive thru. Sometimes we start the fight, it becomes too much for us, we end up letting our fear take control, and our spiral down to the depths of despair is quick and painful.

My life's journey has included a number of frightening, life-threatening crises. Even though I am a fighter and a survivor in dealing with crises, Mr. Hyde continually surfaced to lend his "harmful" hand. Some might say that Mr. Hyde was actually helping in these times of crises. But in actuality, he was ultimately making things worst.

As I shared with you in the first part of this book, I had four major surgeries within a twelve-month period. During that period I gained eighty plus pounds. So not only did I have to deal with these health crises, but the weight I had worked so hard to lose was back causing an added burden on me.

I can never impress on you how deeply I understand this repetitious, destructive pattern because it has been a major downfall for me. Whether dealing with a crisis or not, once I deviate from my diet and take that one taste, have that one non-diet program meal, or that one binge, my dieting effort is done, over, kaput! Then I am quickly submerged in an avalanche of negative thinking, considering myself a failure, and I am flooded with shame, guilt, and self-pity and begin to drown in this sea of negative emotions.

I know that all of you understand this devastating cycle that ruins our progress in a nanosecond. We do not stop to consider the fact that we have been on our diet for three weeks, three months, or for whatever the time period, and we have lost five, ten, or whatever amount of poundage. We do not stop to consider that fact that for those three weeks, or three months, we were doing "it"! We do not consider that we lost inches on our body, are feeling better, looking better, and feeling happier. In a flash, our whole focus immediately becomes one very loud self-judgment: "I am a failure!" Add this component to a current crisis that we are dealing with and it becomes a perfect storm causing a mental and emotional explosion of monumental proportions.

One very important thing to consider when crises arise in our lives is to make ourselves stop (even shout "STOP!" out loud), then ask ourselves these questions: "Will eating this food help my situation, or make things worse for me? Yes, I have to deal with cancer, but won't the weight that I have lost and continue to lose help me in this crisis? Won't staying on my eating plan and doing what is right for my body actually help me to be stronger and deal with this situation better? Will this bag of cookies pay that bill or change my boss's decision?" We know the right answers, yet we have become accustomed to returning to our habit of surrendering to what we have practiced for years, if not decades.

When it does come to crisis, my story is your story, and your story is mine. We understand each other. That is why I wrote this book, and that is why you are reading it. We are one and need to join forces. We are joining forces, now!

We are human beings. Life happens and includes great challenges and crises. We are fighters, survivors, and we can overcome the crises obstacles. Most importantly, we can overcome crisis without losing our control and letting our fears take over. We do this by becoming our own "Crisis Hotline!"

Please remember the desire to change is paramount in the use of these affirmations. You have the power! You are a fighter! You can handle anything! You can and you will survive the crises that comes up in your life!

AFFIRMATIONS ON HANDLING CRISIS

1) I am totally calm during all challenges and create a sense of peace for myself.

2) I effectively manage all challenges and crises and move forward with ease.

3) I always take the proper actions to handle difficult challenges and crisis while maintaining my serenity.

4) Whatever situation arises in my life, I trust my inner guidance, knowing that all is working out for my highest good.

5)   I stop, think logically, and make wise choices to achieve positive results in challenging situations.

6)   I step outside of my comfort zone and handle any challenge or crisis while maintaining my health priorities.

7)   Through any and all challenges or crisis, I choose to remain in a state of peace and love.

AND SO IT IS!

(HUG YOURSELF, REALLY GOOD!)

Chapter Fourteen

On Having Fun

"So I want you to get up now. I want all of you to get up out of your chairs. I want you to get up right now and go to the window. Open it, and stick your head out, and yell, 'I'M AS MAD AS HELL, AND I'M NOT GOING TO TAKE THIS ANYMORE!'" Quote from the screenplay *Network* by Paddy Chayefsky

You know, these are some serious issues that we are dealing with here. It's all about retraining our belief in ourselves, and, yes, it is serious. I am a serious guy, often too serious as I am told by some of my friends. My friends are always telling me to lighten up and have some fun!

So, I want you, all of us, to have some fun. Let's face it, life flies by quicker than we want it to. The time is now. Let's get mad as hell and not take the serious side of life so intensely anymore. Let's have some fun!

We are always extremely focused on losing weight and being perfect on our diets. Though we never-ending dieters make our weight loss the center of our lives, we also have careers, families to take care of, checkbooks to balance, appointments to keep, and all the other countless responsibilities that must be taken care of in our daily living. Sometimes we forget that we need a break and deserve to have some fun.

If it is just to take a drive for a half hour to take in the local sights, do it. Going to a movie or the theater, or just sitting outside and communing with nature, give yourself the time and devote yourself to some of the pleasures that you may have been denying yourself because of that terrifying critical thought process: "I am too fat!" Oh, how I have lived by that thought in the past and I have missed a great deal in my life because of it. I will not allow myself to live that way any longer. I do not want to live that way anymore. Let's be mad as hell and have some fun at last. We all deserve it!

We cannot turn back time, but now is now. Be free, be joyful, and please, have some fun along your path to rediscovering yourself and renewed self-love.

Please remember the desire to change is paramount in the use of these affirmations. You are worthy! You are wonderful! You deserve to treat yourself with kindness! You deserve to have some fun!

AFFIRMATIONS

1) I set aside time in my life to relax and enjoy simple pleasures.

2) I plan my work and play to achieve perfect balance in my life.

3) I allow myself to have fun, laugh out loud, and enjoy the activities and people that bring happiness to me.

4) I nourish myself with the joys of life and it brings me great satisfaction.

5) I allow myself to be secure and confident as I celebrate life with family and friends.

"In all of living, have much fun and laughter.
Life is to be enjoyed, not just endured."
– Gordon B. Hinckley

AND SO IT IS!

(NOW SMILE, AND GIVE YOURSELF A HUGE HUG!)

Chapter Fifteen

The Beginning

"You are on the verge of something magnificent.
Don't give up!"
- Unknown

*I*n every conclusion there is also a beginning. I hope that you have worked consistently with the affirmations and are seeing a change in how you are feeling and living your life. Your job, your family, your friends, and your life are the same, but you are definitely not the same person or doing the same things that you were before using these affirmations. This is your new beginning! This is the realization of your magnificence. I know from my own experience of having worked methodically with the affirmations that I am a different man today than I used to be. My work with the affirmations, as well as sharing them with you in this book, have given me my new beginning, the realization of my true magnificence.

If you have not yet worked with the affirmations, please take time for yourself and make using the affirmations a part of your daily living. Give yourself the time and the chance that you so deserve by using these affirmations as discussed in the introductory chapter of this healing section. You will definitely see how much better you will feel, and you will quickly begin to experience your true magnificence too.

I certainly realize that the ultimate reality for all of us is that we want to lose weight. We are tired of being fat and tired of being never-ending dieters. At some point in our lives, something went amiss and we turned to food. It could have been habits that were formed in our childhoods, a particular life event, a crisis, or an opportunity that led us to food for happiness, to ease our pains or to deal with our fears. Whatever the cause, it ultimately resulted in the development of our crazy relationship with food and diets. Whether it was from our childhood or later in our lives, being fat and dieting became our "Achilles heel" and stayed with us all these years. I really believe that the key to long-term success is, first and foremost, coming to terms with the human healing traits that I have presented in this book.

So where do we go from here? What diet do we pick this time? How do we proceed with getting this weight off and keeping it off? Before we discuss options, the one thing I want you to always remember, is that you are perfect just the way you are, right now, and no matter what you weigh. You are perfect now and always!

As I have expressed before, I know that we are all diet experts to some degree because of our past experiences with dieting. Many of us have acquired so much nutrition education over the years that we could be dietitians and teach the classes. I was talking with a mentor of mine and told him that in the last chapter of my book I was going to include some suggestions about "where we go from here" in regard to dieting. I asked him his suggestions regarding future dieting advice. He said to me, "More than any diet you could suggest, each individual needs to select a program that is a way of life, a permanent change to his or her lifestyle. The program should include a healthy nutrition plan that fits his or her individual needs and life, and gets the weight off healthfully." As soon as I heard his words, I knew that this was sound advice and truthful guidance.

I know the voice in your head (hopefully not as aggressive and loud as before using the affirmations) probably still wants you to seek out that "magic pill." Though this remains a dream of dieters, there is no magic pill. We each need to find our own way, our own nutrition plan or program that offers us a lifestyle that lets us to accomplish our weight loss goals while still allowing us to experience life to its fullest.

We all love success stories. We love to read about the woman who went to her daughter's school and because her daughter was so embarrassed of her mom's weight, she ran away before her classmates knew that the woman was her mother. Being devastated by this event, over the next year the woman lost two hundred pounds. Then there is the story of the man who went to a friend's house and broke a toilet off the wall because of his obesity. He was so overcome with embarrassment and shame, that the realization of his real size finally hit him hard. Over the next year he lost two hundred and fifty pounds by eating only fruits and vegetables. We are thrilled for these people and their stories are great news items, but each of these stories is truly one in a million.

Then we read and see on television the stories of the many individuals who eat nutritionally sound, exercise regularly, and lose an average of five to ten pounds a month. In the period of a year they lose anywhere from fifty to a hundred plus pounds. The difference between these individuals and the "one in a million" news stories is that they lost their weight healthfully while developing a new lifestyle that will allow them to maintain their weight loss and to continue to lose more if necessary. The key word for us here should be "healthfully."

"Bah humbug!" you may exclaim. I totally understand this reaction. I once heard a saying that gives a real wake-up call and is so very true. "The problem is that we think we have the time!" Time passes so quickly. As time passes, we have continued to spin our wheels on diet after diet. Sometimes we start on a diet and "try" to stay on it, convincing ourselves that we actually on a diet when we are in fact continuing our old eating habits while allegedly dieting. Then after a few weeks or months have passed, we either weigh the same or have gained weight while "being on this diet." Many of us have experienced this and know this trick. Then there are those wonderful times when we are really making progress on our diet and then we have that one bite which catapults us into food oblivion as discussed in the chapters on perfectionism and dealing with crises.

The reality is that the time to act is now! I wish I could tell you what and how much to eat, so forth and so on, your weight would drop off quickly, and you would never have to diet again. But unfortunately, I cannot. And, we think we have the time! What if, just what if, we develop a lifestyle of proper eating and exercise (that dreaded word!)? What would happen? Would we lose a pound a week? Two pounds a week? If we're conscientious in our efforts in the development of this new lifestyle, would not these efforts result in a loss of fifty to hundred plus pounds in a year? Well, the answer is, of course, yes! Would this be new territory? Could we do it? It's certainly worth the try, don't you think?

I want to share my recent weight loss journey with you. As I discussed in Chapter Three, after my devastating health issues and the trauma from my four surgeries, I regained eighty plus pounds that I had worked so hard to get off. Now I am losing weight again. By changing my lifestyle with a healthy nutrition program and exercising within my limitations, my weight is coming down, slowly and steadily. Yes, I am still fat, but I am getting lighter and healthier every day. I know without a shadow of a doubt that I would not be losing weight today, or in this manner, if I had not first changed my thought processes and overall vision of the man that I truly am by consistently using the affirmations that I developed and share with you in this book. My journey with these affirmations has changed my life and continues to do so.

What I truly believe for each of you, is with the shifts you are experiencing in your psyche as a result of your affirmation practices, you will accomplish anything you desire including your weight loss goals. But whatever you decide for yourself in regard to diet, I do know this: together we stand, divided we fall! Whatever you decide to do, you do not have to do it alone. Seek out someone, some group, some doctor, or whatever and whomever you can find to help you. I cannot begin to tell you the limitless number of times that I rejoined Weight Watchers® or how many times that I have gone to Overeaters Anonymous® groups over the years. Then there were the therapy groups that I participated in, the very expensive weight loss programs, and all the diet doctors I have seen. Yet the truth is that when I revisit the number of times that I went to a group or participated in a diet program with a group, my success rate was much better than doing it on my own. Again, within this suggestion of seeking help, a program that provides us with an overall long-term lifestyle change is the really the best alternative.

Speaking of not doing it alone, I am here for you. I think that I have shown you through my words that I truly understand you, what you have been through, and what lies ahead. You do not have to do it alone. Please join me on my web site: "My Life as a Diet" (mylifeasadiet.com). I have a blog and there will be much more coming in the future to help us in joining forces to get us where we want to go, that being to live a happy, healthy long life.

The information that I have presented to you here in my book comes from my heart, from the very core of my soul. I know that there are so many of you out there who identify with me. My goals in writing this book are to let you know that you are not alone, that someone out there truly understands you, and that a healing can happen for you if you are willing to make it happen.

My wish for you is only the absolute best in life. I wish for you the best health, the greatest happiness, self-love and acceptance, and the knowledge that at this very moment in time, and with each and every moment that follows, you are perfect in every way, and no matter what you weigh. May your future bring you peace, great happiness, and ultimately an end to your never-ending diets.

AND SO IT SHALL BE...AND SO IT IS!

About the Author

Maurice Horwitz was born and grew up in Houston, Texas, where he still lives today. His education includes a BA in theater arts from the University of Houston, and a MPA master in business from the University of Texas at Austin.

Maurice had hoped to have a career in show business but his journey led him down a completely different path. He became a tax accountant and for the last twenty-six years of his professional career worked for the U.S. Government. With job burn out, Maurice retired early with his intention to dramatically change his life physically, emotionally, and spiritually. The year following his retirement he lost one hundred thirty-eight pounds. The next chapter of Maurice's life led him down a bumpy road that included a number of very serious health crises. During the one-year period of these crises Maurice gained back most of the weight he had recently lost. While recovering from the last of these medical traumas, Maurice realized that his weight and life were totally out of control yet once again. This jolting wake-up call ultimately guided Maurice to develop a life-altering healing plan for his self. With courage and devotion to this plan, Maurice experienced a dramatic change in his psyche and life. He knew the time had arrived to share his deep understanding of living with being fat, never-ending diets, and especially his powerful healing plan to help others like himself. The result of Maurice's work is his book, "My Life As A Diet: Understanding and Healing for Never-ending Dieters!"

This book is for people struggling with weight issues and *"anyone"* wishing to change their life for the better. Maurice shares his simple yet powerful, transformative healing plan giving you the stepping-stones needed to achieve extraordinary results. With personal commitment and a little patience, the plan will guide you to a treasured state of happiness no matter what you weigh or what obstacles that you are facing in your life.

www.ingramcontent.com/pod-product-compliance
Lightning Source LLC
Chambersburg PA
CBHW060908280326
41934CB00007B/1235